Fat and Fertile

Fat and Fertile

How to get pregnant
in a bigger body

Nicola Salmon

This book is dedicated to every person who has been made to feel worth less because of their body.

About the Author

Nicola is a fat-positive and feminist fertility coach. She advocates for change in how fat women are treated on their fertility journey. She supports fat women (and others with disordered eating) who are struggling to get pregnant to find peace with their body, find their own version of health and finally escape the yo-yo dieting cycle.

Nicola is a qualified Fertility Coach, Acupuncturist and Naturopath. She initially trained to be a Clinical Scientist at King's College Hospital, London with a masters in Medical Engineering and Physics, before life took a strange turn and she was diagnosed with Post Traumatic Stress Disorder. Nicola eventually found acupuncture was able to support her and she was so intrigued by how it worked that she spent four years training to be an Acupuncturist and Naturopath.

As Nicola was diagnosed with PCOS at 16, she was drawn to treating hormonal conditions and fertility. After starting her own family, Nicola started down the long path to making peace with food and her body and realised that people in bigger bodies were being completely discriminated against, with regards to fertility support.

Nicola now advocates for people in bigger bodies to receive the treatment that they are entitled to. She has written for *The Metro*, *Scary Mommy*, *The UnEdit*, *Fertility Road* and other publications.

Table of Contents

Acknowledgements

I will forever be grateful for all the people who have come before me and risked their lives to fight the injustices that people face because of the body that they were born into.

To all the people who are doing this work right now and sharing their gifts with me and the world. You have such a profound impact on my life, whether you know it or not! Without you, my life would be so much poorer. Here are some of the incredible people I'd like to thank who share their work tirelessly.

Abby Wasik, Alice Connolly, Amanda Hayden, Amanda Laird, Amanda Martinez Beck, Amber Marshall, Amy Hanneke, Angela Meadows, Ashlee Bennett, Brianna M. Campos, Cara Cifelli, Cara Harbstreet, Caroline Dooner, Chelsea Karcher, Christy Harrison, Dana Falsetti, Dana Sturtevant, Dani Adriana, Elyse Resch, Evelyn Tribole, Fiona Willer, Hayley McLean, Hilary Kinavey, Holly Grigg-Spall, Ilya from Decolonizing Fitness, Jen McLellan, Jes Baker, Jessi Haggerty, Jessica Campbell, Jodie Mitchell, Julie Duffy Dillon, Kamilla Møller Rasmussen, Kat Stroud, Kathleen Meehan, Kelly Diels, Kimmie Singh, Kirsten Ackerman, Laura Dennison, Laura Thomas, Lily Nichols, Linda Bacon, Linn Thorstensson, Lucy Aphramor, Maddie Deakin, Maria Paredes, Meg Boggs, Megan Jayne Crabbe, Melissa A. Fabello, Meredith Noble, Mia O'Malley, Michelle Elman, Nicole McDermid, Rachel Foy, Ragen Chastain, Robyn Nohling, Sofie Hagen, Sonalee Rashatwar, Sonya Renee Taylor, Stephanie Yeboah, Summer Innnen, Terri Waters, Tiffany Roe, Tonya Beauchaine, Tracy Vazquez, Victoria Welsby, Virgie Tovar, Virginia Sole-Smith, Whitney Blakeslee, Whitney Catalona

To the phenomenal people who run the charity, AnyBody. I have known you all for such a short time, but I already feel like I'm home.

To all my friends in my life who have loved me even when I didn't love myself: Rosie Allston, Sian Redwood, Charlotte Riley, Angharad Fletcher, Rhian Bird, Katie Bardsley, Usha Deering, Nicola Haggett and all my inspiring friends at CrossFit 2012.

To all my wonderful business buddies who have supported me in growing and shaping my business., Elizabeth Buckley-Goddard, Ann Merle Feldman, Laura Agar Wilson, Lisa Lister, Lauren Gayfer, Fabiana Nilsson and Natalie Silverman.

To all my clients and supporters who have allowed me to be a small part of their journey to becoming incredible parents.

And finally to my loving family: My husband Paul, who supports my dreams everyday. My two beautiful boys, Sebby and Isaac, who finally showed me how harmful dieting was to my life. My wonderful parents, Sandra and Martin, who taught me how to love unconditionally. My sister Sarah, who has been my partner in crime since she could walk. My incredible Mother-in-law Wendy, sister-in-law Alison and all our extended family.

Introduction

If you are in a bigger body and want to become a parent, the chances are that you have faced some problems. Maybe your doctor has dismissed your request for help and told you to "just lose weight." Maybe your friends and family have taken you aside and told you that they are concerned for your health. Maybe all you can think about is how you need to be healthier before you can become a mother.

After all, we are told time and time again that fat is unhealthy. We have been led to believe that getting pregnant when fat is a sin worse than death. There are so many myths around getting pregnant in a fat body.

Myth One - Getting pregnant will be impossible for you when you are in a larger body.

Myth Two - If you are lucky enough to get to past that first hurdle, then your pregnancy will be riddled with risks and illnesses that are caused by being fat.

Gestational diabetes, miscarriage, babies that are too big, high blood pressure - all problems that people in fat bodies are told to expect.

Myth Three - And once you've had your baby? Well, then your child is more likely to be at risk of a host of other problems.

So why on earth would you not want to lose weight? If this was the truth, if this is what the research shows, why would anyone get pregnant in a fat body?

Introduction

I got pregnant in a fat body. Twice. The first time I was eaten up with guilt throughout my whole pregnancy. I planned to lose weight before I got pregnant, but you see, I thought I had time. I was told getting pregnant was going to be impossible for me, (myth one) so I thought I would have at least a year to find yet another diet to help me lose weight.

But my husband and I got pregnant quickly, and after the initial shock wore off, I was terrified. At first, I thought I had an ectopic pregnancy. Before each scan, I convinced myself that I was going to have a miscarriage. I was sure that I had gestational diabetes and that I would need a c section because my baby was too big. None of that came true. I had a completely unremarkable pregnancy (myth two). So why was I so worried at every turn? I truly believed that I didn't deserve this pregnancy and baby because I was fat.

This book is for you if you've ever felt that way and felt ashamed to tell people that you want to get pregnant because of your size.

This book is for you if you are terrified of talking to your doctor about getting pregnant or have had a horrific experience when you did.

This book is for you if you are looking for support in getting pregnant and have no idea where to turn next.

The truth is that support and resources beyond the "lose weight" advice is few and far between. In our culture, weight is seen as controllable. Most people believe that you could lose weight if you wanted to. We are told that if the diet fails, it is us that have failed. We weren't motivated enough or strict enough. We didn't have the will power to follow through, and that is a failing on our part.

But there is **ONE big assumption** that we are making here. That we can control our weight. There is a considerable body of research that shows that diets fail. It's not us that fails, diets fail. We know to the same confidence level that we know that smoking causes lung cancer that restrictive diets do not work in the long term for 90%+ of people.

Take a deep breath and let that sink in. Diets do not work.

Every single weight loss strategy you took part in, set you up to fail. It was not your fault that you couldn't lose weight or maintain a weight deemed acceptable. You did not fail those diets. Those diets failed you.

People are profiting from this need that has been placed upon us to look a certain size. The dieting industry is worth $70 billion in the US alone. Do you think we would need to spend this extortionate amount of money on diets if they worked?

Now I know you are probably going to be going through a whole heap of emotions right now, I know I did when I discovered this information. You might be feeling angry at the appalling way that we are being exploited by society. You might be in total disbelief and denial ready to throw this book straight in the bin. You might be rocked to the core with sadness and grief at all the time and energy spent chasing the unicorn of a perfect body, which never really existed.

Above all, you might feel hopeless. If you were told weight loss was your only option, and here I am telling you that weight loss is impossible, what the hell are you supposed to do now?

Stay with me, my love. In this book, I am going to share my story and show you the steps I take with my clients to move away from the scales and towards a healthy and happy pregnancy.

The biggest thing you can do right now is to show yourself some kindness. You cannot control what has happened in the past. You did your absolute best with what you knew at the time, and that is all anyone can ask.

You've got this, my love.

Note about language

Through my journey, I have come to self-identify as fat. There are lots of words used to describe bigger bodies - fat, obese, overweight and plus size are the most common ones.

Some of these words are very problematic. Obese is the medicalised term identifying being fat as an illness and overweight implies that you are not a "normal" weight.

Many fat activists have worked tirelessly to embrace the descriptor fat as on it's own it means that you have a fat body, nothing more, nothing less. It is only because we have added meaning to what being fat means in our society that being fat is something to be avoided.

The word fat can be triggering if you have been bullied and abused with it so be gentle with yourself, but I would love to you to begin to question the language you use around your own body and how it benefits you.

Throughout the book, I use the word "woman/women" to identify people in bodies who have uteri, ovaries and vaginas and want to get pregnant in their body. I understand that not all people with a uterus identify with this word. This book is for all people with a uterus who want to become pregnant.

Chapter 1 - How to stop trying to lose weight

This book was nearly never written.

Not because I'm not passionate about fertility and helping fat women.Not because fat women who want to get pregnant can't be helped. But because of me. I put off writing this book for over two years after I had decided to write it. Why? Because I was worried that if I wrote a book about being fat that it meant I would be fat forever. If I became the fat fertility coach, then being fat would be part of who I am and I would never be able to lose weight and therefore never be healthy and happy because it's been so entrenched in me that my worth is based on my weight.

I was too frightened to write this book because, in the end, it would mean I would never be happy. But what I came to realise was that I was completely wrong. It's not about what the weighing scales say. It's not about what your BMI is or how much fat you can measure around your waist.

By focusing on weight loss, we are perpetuating the story that women have to be a certain size to be healthy. We are continuing the myth that women are on this planet to look pretty and do as we're told. We do not have to accept that as our reality anymore.

So if you've picked this book up in the hope that it is (yet another) diet aimed at helping you lose weight to get pregnant, put it down again. But if you have an inkling that maybe, just maybe, losing weight is entirely the wrong thing to focus on when you're trying to get pregnant, then read on. Together we are going to unravel how you can get pregnant in a fat body and how this is going to change your entire life for the better.

Weight loss isn't the answer

If you have ever looked at the research surrounding getting pregnant in a fat body, you will have been terrified. There are papers upon papers that show that the higher your BMI[1], the more problems you face conceiving.

What you might not know is that there is also lots of research that shows that diets are not evidence-based medicine. Every time a doctor has asked you to lose weight, there has been little to no evidence that shows that losing weight will improve your condition or symptoms.

That's not to say that your doctors are trying to trick you. The evidence available shows that people with higher BMIs experience more problems in all areas of their health, including fertility, so why is this not the same thing?

The evidence shows that the higher your BMI, the higher your risks of ill health. This is not the same as showing that weight loss improves your condition. Jessica Campbell of Body Balance Nutrition and the Instagram account @haes_studentdoctor did some digging into the research and found that even though many doctors state that just a 5% weight loss can improve fertility, there are no published dose-response studies demonstrating a relationship between weight loss and fertility. I.e. there are no studies that show if you lose X kg, then your chance of getting pregnant increases by X%.

---

[1] BMI stands for Body Mass Index. BMI is a standard measure used in healthcare based on your height and weight. BMI has been wholly debunked as a meaningful indicator of health. BMI has no meaning when applied to individual health, as it was designed to look at trends in population health. You can learn more about BMI in some of the books I recommend in the Further Reading section at the back of the book.

Weight loss efforts often incorporate health-promoting behaviours such as drinking more water, eating more vegetables, moving your body more. These health-promoting behaviours may improve your condition, but that is very different than the weight loss improving your health.

In Linda Bacon's book "Health At Every Size", they started a revolution to highlight that healthy habits are far more valuable to our health than our BMI could ever be. The book started the HAES movement worldwide and the movement promotes social justice and support for people of all sizes. Finding practitioners who are aware of and align with the HAES principles can be so powerful for your health.

Although BMI and increased health issues increase together, this is a correlation, i.e. as one goes up, the other goes up. This is NOT causation; one is causing the other thing to happen. There is no evidence that fat causes health problems. Correlation is not causation. The reason that this correlation exists is based on two factors that are not taken into account during research for fat people.

Weight Bias

The first of these two factors is called weight bias and is something you have likely experienced yourself if you live in a fat body. Weight bias means that if you are over a certain weight, there is a bias against you. Maybe you thought you were the only one who felt judged about your body after seeing your doctor? You may have blamed yourself and put it down to feeling "too sensitive". I promise you; you are not alone.

This is how weight bias works. Our healthcare professionals live in the same world that we do and are immersed in the same diet culture, where fat is bad and thin is best. When they train, they are taught that people in bigger bodies experience higher risks of serious illnesses, eat crap foods and don't look after their bodies.

We go and visit our doctor. They look at our body and tell us that we need to lose weight. No matter the reason we went in, the problem is our bodies and our weight. If we are lucky, they will say it kindly and offer us the latest dieting advice. If we are not so lucky, we will be mocked and shamed and leave the room in tears.

These visits cause two big problems, aside from the biggest problem of all, severely damaging our mental health. The first problem is that it leads to fat people avoiding their healthcare professionals. When you are made to feel like crap, it will take severe symptoms and desperation ever to want to go back there. The second problem is a delay in diagnosis from your doctor. If you are turned away and told to lose weight, it will probably be another six months before your doctor will perform diagnostic tests and find the root cause of your actual issue.

Both these problems lead to considerable delays in appropriate healthcare treatment for people in fat bodies. So guess what? These people have higher incidences of serious illnesses. Not because of the fat on their body, but because their diagnosis and treatment have been delayed and therefore their prognosis is worse. This is a scary thing to realise. But it's even more reason to begin to advocate for yourself with your doctors. To not shy away from the difficult conversations about your health and to expect respect from other human beings. See "Chapter 5 - How to advocate for your fat body" for more support with this.

Weight cycling

The second reason why BMI and health risks increase is to do with our old friend yo-yo dieting. So many women in larger bodies have been yo-yo dieting since before puberty. Going on increasingly restrictive diets over the years as the diets become less and less effective and their weight increases.

What impact does the constant restriction of calories have on our bodies? What impact does our weight constantly moving up and down have on our hormones and our fertility? The continuous weight increase and decrease are called weight cycling, and there is a considerable body of research that shows that weight cycling alongside weight bias causes higher risks for people in bigger bodies.

You cannot blame fat for the issues we see in the fertility world. There is a much bigger picture of the health of a fat woman than the inches of fat you see around her middle. But if you're reading this thinking: but that's me. I've yo-yo dieted my whole life. Have a ruined my fertility? Am I putting my pregnancy and unborn baby at risk if I try to get pregnant?

The great news is that the human body has an incredible capacity for healing. As soon as you move away from the utterly unnatural way that we have been treating our body through restrictive diet and punishing exercise, you are giving your body the chance to heal. You can literally change the way that your DNA expresses itself in your body through your actions and create an environment where you can have a healthy body, a healthy pregnancy and a healthy baby.....in your fat body.

Diets don't work

A diet is any form of eating where there is restriction involved. This goes way beyond joining a weight loss club or following a particular diet online. Diets are sneaky, and they can be found in many places where you might not think to look.

Can't eat a particular food group? That's a diet.
Can't eat at certain times. That's a diet.
Can't eat two types of food together? Diet.
Clean dieting? Diet

So many of the new wellness trends are just diets in disguise. Any form of eating where you are following rules or external cues for what you eat or are trying to lose weight is a diet. Any time where you are demonising particular food groups or basing your worth on how well you can follow a way of eating is a diet.

Whenever we go on a diet, the physical and mental impact on our health far outweighs any benefits from the health-promoting behaviours we may follow on the diet. I'm not going to be diving into all the details about that research in this book. There are lots more books out already doing a great job of explaining the research behind this. You can find more resources in the further reading section at the back of this book, but right now I recommend grabbing the free e-book "Everything You've Been Told About Weight Loss Is Bullshit" by Louise Adams, MAPS and Fiona Willer, APD.[2]

In their e-book, Adams and Willer explain that "2-5 years after dieting, 95% of dieters are back to where they started, and about one to two thirds of people end up heavier than they were before they began! This fact is SO well known that it's included as "Level A" evidence (meaning it's the highest level of evidence possible in science) from the Australian National Health & Medical Research Council."

There are no diets that will give you sustained weight loss without weight regain beyond two to five years. I know what you're thinking. You know this friend of a friend who did this diet. She lost so much weight and is still thin five

---

[2] You can download "Everything You've Been Told About Weight Loss Is Bullshit" at https://dietingisbs.carrd.co/

years later. The question I want to ask you is "But at what cost?" What continually restricting rules is she setting herself around eating? How is she punishing herself with exercise every day to maintain that weight loss? This is the reality for so many women. We are told that we have to be constantly policing our bodies and our food intake to stay small.

When I read all the research behind diets, I wasn't surprised that they don't work, and I doubt that you're surprised either. This has been the reality of my life for the past 20 years. Why do we believe that we'll be healthier and happier when we are thinner? The world is built for thin people. People in fat bodies are seen as an anomaly and aren't taken into consideration when creating our environment. It is much harder to navigate the world in a fat body, and the fatter your body is, the harder it becomes.

I would describe myself as living in a small fat body. I can sometimes buy clothes on the high street, although the process is very triggering and the selection is often tiny. When I navigate public transport, I can squeeze my body into the seats, but that isn't the case for many people in bigger bodies.

It can be hard to go on an aeroplane in their ever-decreasing sized seats.
It can be impossible to find clothes that fit your body comfortably.
It can be challenging to navigate a shop with narrow aisles.

Simple things that people in small bodies don't even think about can become impossible for people in bigger bodies.

What do you really want when you say that you want to lose weight?

Maybe you want to be able to live your life without having to think about if your body size is going to be an issue. Maybe you want healthcare that's not based on your size, but based on the actual health of your body. Maybe you want to feel healthier, stronger, more confident in your body? You want to get pregnant.

I want you to challenge your thinking. The things that you think you will get from losing weight, the ways that you want to feel in your body. How many of them can you get right now, in the body that you're in?

Exercise

So let's get started. What things are you putting off for when you get skinny?

- Maybe it's a new job you only think you'll get when you have more confidence (aka a thinner body).
- Maybe you'll finally be able to wear clothes that feel like you.
- Maybe you want to take up some sports or new hobbies but are afraid of what people will think of you.
- Maybe just maybe you are putting off really trying to get pregnant until you are more healthy (aka society's version of healthy).
Grab a pen and paper or download the "Fat and Fertile" accompanying PDF that contains all the exercises from the book that you can fill in straight on your computer or print off.

Access the PDF at nicolasalmon.co.uk/bookbonus

Write a list. What things would you do differently if you were thin?

Write down at least ten things although I'm sure you've got a list as long as your arm of things that you've been putting off.

Now take a long hard look at the list.

What things can you physically not do because of your fat? Label them A

What things are you not doing because you don't really believe you could do them. Label them B

What things are you doing because of what others might think? Label them C

Any other random excuses label D

Lots of Bs and Cs I bet!!

Your limiting beliefs about your body and about what other people think is holding you back (little secret- most people are so wrapped up in their own stuff that they probably aren't thinking about you)
What's the one thing on that list that you really want to do? What's the biggie?

How are you going to make that happen now? No ifs or buts. What do you need to do to make this thing happen in the next week? What action can you take today to get you one step closer to this goal? Your life is happening right now, with or without you. Don't let it pass you by because of what people might be thinking.

How to stop trying to lose weight

Now onto that, pesky thought about needing to be healthier to get pregnant. Do you know what this is? It's your fat phobia in disguise. Healthier usually is code for skinnier. It is disguised as a helpful suggestion. We are all supposed to be healthy to get pregnant, right? Getting healthier is the responsible thing to do, the grown-up thing to do. Except that getting healthier is not your real intention.

Being healthy looks different for everyone. Being healthy means doing things that feel good for your body. Choosing foods that make you feel vibrant. Laughing. Moving in a way that makes you feel alive. Being healthy does not mean being thin and being fat does not mean you are unhealthy.

Every "get healthy" endeavour I ever made (until 2018) was a disguised attempt to lose weight. No matter what I told everyone else, I intended to get skinny so that it would be socially acceptable to society. Even now I'm not immune from this. Recently I've started CrossFit, a functional movement class combining gymnastics, weight lifting, and metabolic conditioning.

Let me paint you a picture. I was the chubby girl, panting in last place at cross country. I was the little girl shouted at ballet class because I couldn't sit on the floor, put my feet together and touch the floor with my knees. I couldn't climb the rope in gym class, and I never played sport out of choice. Exercise was not my strong suit.

For the first time, I've chosen to exercise to feel strong and look after my body. Hand on heart, my intention is to take the best care that I can of this body. But the thoughts still cross my mind…. Ooo am I starting to get skinnier? Maybe I'll be able to buy a whole new wardrobe in three months…. I wonder what my friends will say …. I regularly fell into that daydream of the weight loss transformation that everyone chases.

Then I have to snap myself out of it. That's not why I'm doing this. Be honest with yourself about your motivation and your intention. Are you trying to get healthy to lose weight? Are you trying to lose weight to get pregnant? The biggest question of all is, how have we strayed so far away from automatically making the healthiest choices for us? Regardless of our size, regardless of whether we are trying to get pregnant? Why isn't our motivation to take the best care of our bodies that we are able?

I have a few choice words to say about our culture, the advertisers, the patriarchy. But we still have a choice, and you can choose, today, to change paths. To begin to think about what the best thing for you is. The best thing for your body, the best thing for your mind and the best thing for your whole wellbeing? Because what's best for you is what's best for baby.

The effects of dieting

Now if you've been around the dieting block once or twice, I'm sure you'll be aware of all the big diets out there. The diet industry is worth $70 billion in the US alone. The big question is how it is sustainable? If the diets work, then why are we still fat? These programs create and maintain eating disorders. That's the blunt truth. The diet industry wants to keep us fat.

When you are on a diet, when you are restricting your food intake based on calories or points or syns or whatever fancy new term they use, you are creating a disordered pattern around food. You are no longer listening to your internal cues. When you are using language that creates a hierarchy around food you eat, you have a disordered eating issue.

Do you have "good foods" and "bad foods"? Do you "treat yourself" to food? Were you "naughty" the other day when you had a doughnut? It's not your fault. The language and the culture we have grown up in around food has contributed to this massively and should not be underestimated, but the diet industry is now intensifying these issues for pure profit. I'm sure these phrases will be very familiar to you.

"I've fallen off the wagon."

"I'll start again on Monday."

"I've failed now so I might as well eat this whole bar of chocolate and start again in the morning."

Who invented this so-called wagon? I'll let you in on a little secret .... there is no wagon. Your worth as a human does not depend on what food you put in your mouth. Your worthiness to be a mother does not depend on the number on those scales. I know it is tempting to keep trying to lose the weight and then you'll feel happy and healthy. I know that you think losing the weight will solve all your problems. That is the story we are fed time and time again. Every time you see another before and after picture, you think that could be me.

But this is the problem: When you start dieting with the intention of losing weight as fast as you can, you are punishing your body. To lose weight quickly, you are told to drastically reduce the calories or portions you are eating, exercise to an extreme degree or both. Both of these actions put your body under a lot of stress.

Reducing your calories significantly signals to your body that there is a famine, that there is not enough food available in your environment right now. After all, that is the only reason your food intake would've reduced in our ancestor's time. Your body instinctually diverts resources away from your reproductive system. If there were a famine, it would be an awful time to get pregnant for both you and baby. Your body is protecting you and keeping you safe.

The same goes for exercise. Excessive exercise signals to your body that you are in danger. In our ancestor's time, we would be running away from predators, and the continued stress of exercise on our bodies puts them into fight or flight response. The body primes the muscles, lungs and cardiovascular systems to move and shuts off digestion and reproduction. Again this is to ensure your survival and keep you safe.

Our bodies have not yet caught up with our 21st-century living. It doesn't understand the difference between famine and dieting or survival and triathlons. The tools we are using to improve our health are hindering our fertility. I hear that exasperated sigh. I know what you're thinking. WFT man!?!!! You've been doing this stuff your whole freaking life to try and reach this unobtainable goal. You've been doing everything you've been told, and it's still not good enough!

You've always been good enough. But now it's time to do things your way. It's time to listen to what your body needs and to heal your relationship with food and with your body. As they say, it's the only one you've got.

What would it mean if you stayed exactly as you are?

Let me ask you a question, what would happen if you stayed exactly the same weight as you are now? How would you feel? What would it mean? When I first asked myself this question, my first feeling was panic! Shit! I thought if I stayed this size forever, what would I do? What does it really mean to be a fat woman, not trying to lose weight?

This was a completely alien concept as my whole identity has been based on being a fat woman trying to lose weight my entire life. It's the only vaguely socially acceptable way to live as a fat woman if you are at least trying to lose weight. You need to be able to spout off the latest way to are trying to get thin.

How to stop trying to lose weight

What would it mean just to be a fat woman? I would buy clothes that fit me and look good now, instead of buying some that were slightly too small to "motivate" myself to lose weight. I would stop wasting so much energy on thinking about what foods to eat and how to move my body. There'd be no point if I were going to stay the same size. Instead of choosing what to eat and how to move my body based on what's going to make me skinnier, I would choose food and movement that make me feel good.

I would be free to do other things with all the excess energy I'd been wasting on losing weight. Think of all the minutes/hours/days you've wasted worrying about what food to eat, feeling guilty about the food you've already eaten and planning how you were going to lose weight. All that time in the future is now free to do epic things. Maybe you could learn a new language, do something creative, change the world - the possibilities of what you can do are endless.

Instead of focusing on losing weight to get pregnant, I would focus on making my body as healthy as possible to get pregnant. The thought that I'm too fat to get pregnant wouldn't even cross my mind. After all, your weight wouldn't be in your ability to change.

Doesn't that sound incredible?

Doesn't that sound a million times less stressful way to live? And all it takes is a mindset shift. You are moving away from focusing on losing weight to focusing on nourishing and loving your body now. Of course, that doesn't necessarily mean you're going to stay the same size forever, but when you start to make decisions about your health and wellbeing from a place of love and nourishment, your body can only get healthier and happier.

Your size is entirely irrelevant to the conversation.

So what does that mean in the real world when you want to get pregnant?

It means that you can experiment with food (there is no good food and bad food - those are just labels that we've put on food) and find what works best for your body. Notice how food makes you feel, how it affects your mood, your energy, your digestive system, your sleep. Food can affect every part of your body, so begin to notice what foods make you feel great and what foods make you feel like crap.

Once you have this information, you can make informed decisions about what food you want to eat. That doesn't mean you never eat food that makes you feel crap, it means that you think - "yeah I'm going to feel a bit crap eating this food, but it tastes delicious, and that's what I choose right now for my mental health." It's a choice, and it's hard to make that choice when you have no idea what effect the food has on you. Your body is intelligent, and when you start to listen, you will know what foods your body needs and what it doesn't. You'll begin to notice when you feel hungry and when you are eating for other reasons like when you feel sad, angry or bored.

This is the foundation of a concept called Intuitive Eating. You can read more about this in "Intuitive Eating" Evelyn Tribole and Elyse Resch and "Just Eat It" by Dr Laura Thomas.

The fear is that you won't be able to control yourself around food. You've been taught that you can't be trusted with food, that you will eat and eat and eat until you make yourself sick. It's a choice. When you choose you to love your body now and look after it the best that you can, that behaviour will eventually not even occur to you. We know that bingeing is a biological response to starvation and deprivation. When you deprive yourself of foods and the energy that your body needs, it works so hard to survive and ensures that all you can think about is getting high-calorie food in your mouth ASAP.

How to stop trying to lose weight

Maybe the biggest obstacle you'll encounter is others that are very uncomfortable with how you're choosing to live your life. They are uncomfortable because this thinking flies in the face of everything they've been taught. It shakes the foundations on which everything they know and believe about themselves lies on.

Jes Baker calls this "body currency". In her blog post "Why People hate Tess Munster (and other happy fat people)", she describes so eloquently why happy fat people are seen as such a problem.

"It goes like something this: we are taught as a society that IF we achieve the ideal body that we see in traditional media (and not before) we will then obtain love, worthiness, success and ultimately- happiness. Which is what we all want, right?

Because the vast majority of our culture buys into this, we have millions upon millions of people **investing everything they have** into achieving this ultimate goal. The goal being- thinness which *obviously* equals happiness, remember? (Note: other body "goals" also apply here, like able bodied/lighter skin color/ cisgender appearance etc.) SO, they spend their lives in a perpetual state of self-loathing (its called inspiration!) while working their asses off to become that ideal. We, as Americans, sink billions of dollars into beauty products every year. Between the millions of us on diets, we gift the weight loss industry and other weight loss products over $60 billion dollars as well. 14 million of us had cosmetic procedures in 2012 and yes, that number keeps growing. Perhaps we starve ourselves or maybe we just fixate on our calorie count like it determines our salvation. Maybe we make the gym our god. Whatever we choose individually, we as a country have made 'fixing our bodies' our main obsession and we let it consume our life. This happens for most of us whether we choose to acknowledge it or not. We live to give the quest towards impossible perfection (marketed as happiness) our all.

So THEN after all of this, when a fat chick- who *hasn't* done the work, who *hasn't* tried to fix her body, who *doesn't* have any interest in the gospel we so zealously believe in, *stands up and says*: I'M HAPPY! ...we freak the fuck out.

Because: that bitch just broke the rules. She just cut in front of us in line. She just unwittingly ripped us off. And she essentially made our lifetime of work totally meaningless."[3]

When you change the game, it freaks people out. All of a sudden, they begin to question their choices, their beliefs, and their thoughts, and that's scary. You know that though because that's what we are doing here. Maybe they are ready for the change, or perhaps they're not. Either way, it's not your job to change them. It's not your job to convince them that your way is right and their way is wrong. You cannot change others. The only thing you're in charge of is your thoughts and actions. They might try and change you because you're making them feel so bloody awkward. They might shame you into thinking that your body isn't capable of getting pregnant (it is). They might make rude comments or snide remarks or talk about you behind your back. They might tell you what you eat or what you should or shouldn't wear.

In their own way, they are trying to help. Rightly or wrongly, they are trying to help you conform to our societies standards of what you should look like to be healthy and get pregnant. That doesn't mean you have to listen.

Acknowledge that they mean well but tell them to mind their own business. Be confident in the fact that every decision you're making is the best decision for your health, wellbeing and future family. Only you can make these decisions because only you know your body. Only you know the consequences of the

---

[3] You can find the full blog post at http://www.themilitantbaker.com/2015/01/why-people-hate-tess-munster-and-other.html and read Jes' books, "Things No-one Will Tell Fat Girls" and "Landwhale: On Turing Insults Into Nicknames, Why Body Image Is Hard, and How Diets Can Kiss My Ass".

foods you eat, the way you move, the thoughts you think, and how you spend your time. The power is yours. So it's time to switch your thinking.

Exercise

Grab a pen and paper or download the "Fat and Fertile" accompanying PDF that contains all the exercises from the book that you can fill in straight on your computer or print off. Access the PDF at nicolasalmon.co.uk/bookbonus

Copy out the below words and sign the declaration.

I ……..[insert your name]….. accept my body for exactly the way it is.

Every decision I make for my body will be one that nurtures me in some way. That will look different at different times, but I accept that my health and my body will change over my cycle and over the years.

I choose not to compare what my health looks like with others.

I choose to love my body unconditionally as I know that it is doing its best to keep me alive. I will trust that it knows best and listen to each sign and symptom so that I can learn to nourish it in the best possible way.

I choose to believe that my body is capable of incredible things, including getting pregnant, having a healthy pregnancy and giving birth to a healthy baby.

I am doing the best that I can at this moment, and that is enough.

With love forever

……..[sign your name]………..

Chapter 2 - Fertility support for fat people

Going to the doctor as a fat person is a big deal. If you are living in a fat body, I'm sure you have some stories to tell about the poor treatment you have faced from medical professionals. Even if you can't think of any huge traumas, I bet you can think of many times when your weight was blamed for a completely unrelated illness, when your doctor assumed things about your diet and lifestyle based on your size or when you've felt completely ashamed when leaving the doctors office.

Most people wait 6-12 months of trying naturally to get pregnant before seeing their doctor. If you have already been to see your doctor with fertility questions, I hope that you got referred for some basic hormone tests and received some support. Sadly, this is not the case for most women. The typical story I hear from my clients is that they are told to come back in another 6-12 months once they've lost weight. No blood tests ordered. No questions about their diet or lifestyle. No basic health tests like blood pressure taken. The doctor wrongly assumes based on the body they see before them, that the person is unhealthy and cannot get pregnant due to their size.

If you're fat and go to the doctors seeking help to get pregnant, you will be told to lose weight. There is no doubt in the minds of doctors and researchers that losing weight will improve your chances of getting pregnant. Knowing what you know how, about how losing weight using diets is impossible and how fat isn't even the problem, you can see how completely messed up this system is.

Women are being made to feel utterly ashamed of their bodies for the fact that they are fat, and they cannot get pregnant. They are made to feel that it is 100% their fault that they cannot lose weight, even though we know that it's impossible to lose weight on diets and that the fact that they cannot get pregnant has nothing to do with their size.

Body size is typically categorised using Body Mass Index (BMI). BMI is a basic measure based on your weight and height, which spits out a number. This number will tell you if you are "underweight" "normal" "overweight" "obese" and "morbidly obese." BMI was actually created to look at health trends in large groups of people, it was never intended or designed to be applied to individuals, so how are we now in a position where this number is being used to decide who is eligible for fertility support including IVF?

A BMI of 30 is often given as a threshold for basic testing and fertility support, but even women under this threshold are not immune to being shamed for their body size. If you've been given a label on the BMI scale, throw it out! It's bloody useless. It's time to start looking at your health differently. It's not about the numbers on the scale, on the tape measure or a chart. It's about how you feel when you wake up, how much energy you have and how happy you feel on a daily basis.

I live in the UK, and our healthcare is provided by the National Health Service (NHS). The NHS are given recommendations of what to provide as a service, but this is hugely determined by money and funding. The National Institute for Health and Care Excellence (NICE– the agency that provides national guidance and advice about healthcare) states that every woman in the U.K. under 40 should have access to 3 rounds of IVF if they have not been able to have a baby after two years of unprotected sex.

In the guidelines, they state that:

Fertility support for fat people

"Women should be informed that female BMI should ideally be in the range 19–30 before commencing assisted reproduction, and that a female BMI outside this range is likely to reduce the success of assisted reproduction procedures."

These guidelines themselves are based upon biased research into weight and fertility, but it's important to highlight that they are not restricting access to treatment based on BMI. It's up to individual areas to decide how to spend their budget. In most areas the available funding is one cycle at best – some don't offer any at all. This is a diabolical situation with couples being forced to sell their car, remortgage their houses and wrack up huge credit card bills to have a baby. Don't even get me started on the extortionate charges from many IVF clinics in the UK.

Another criteria placed on access to fertility treatment in the majority of areas is a BMI limit of 30. This is not a limit set by the NICE guidelines and the evidence that a BMI of 30 as a suitable restriction is insufficient. Private clinics in the UK also often pick an arbitrary BMI number as a barrier to fertility treatment. A BMI of 35 seems to be the maximum BMI for the majority of clinics. BMI gives no meaningful indication to the health of the individual and her likelihood of IVF being successful.

Research in 2010[4] showed that there was very limited evidence to support any of the arguments used to restrict IVF based on size.

They found insufficient evidence that shows any relationship between high BMI and reduced birth rates. They also saw no significant difference in miscarriage rates or other pregnancy complications with a high BMI.

Furthermore, none of this evidence begins to unravel the weight cycling and weight stigma faced by these women.

_____

[4] https://academic.oup.com/humrep/article/25/4/815/700269

Nicola Salmon

The emphasis on BMI to determine your health is misleading.

Take me, for example.

I would describe my experience as a fat woman as being typical. I started being aware of food and dieting before puberty. I have been on upwards of 20 different diets, losing weight, then gaining even more weight. Spending all my time, energy and money focused on trying to become a socially acceptable size. I stopped eating fat, cut out the carbs, joined the gym, did a juice detox, tried the shakes, severely restricted my calories and portions, punished my body with exercise. Let me make this clear. This is normal for a fat woman to go through. I would go as far as to say that the majority of women in the western world experience this to some degree.

57% of women in the UK have been on a diet in the past year. This is what's messed up our fertility — the unrealistic expectations placed on us to be a certain size, to look a certain way. I am a very intelligent young(ish) woman, but I've spent my whole life obsessed with food. How can you account for that in a study? It's not that women are fat; it's that society has created a culture where these women have had to put their body through extreme circumstances to try and fit in. But they still blame themselves for not being able to lose weight.

The picture in the rest of the world sadly isn't much different. Fertility clinics all over the world use BMI to restrict access to fertility treatment.

What if I need to access treatment?

It's completely understandable if you still feel you have to lose weight after reading this. After all, if you cannot get pregnant naturally and need fertility support, the system is set up so that you have to lose weight to access the treatment.

If you are able, find a doctor or clinic who can support you at your current size. They do exist, although they can be hard to come by. Research each clinic that you may be able to use. Find out what their policies are around supporting people of size.

If you are unable to switch doctor or clinic for whatever reason and need to lose weight to get treatment, please do not feel guilty. It is your body, and it is your choice. It is, however, important to fully understand the risks and benefits when you make your decision about what to do.

Benefits of losing weight for fertility treatment

Access fertility treatment that you need
Reduction in weight bias faced by medical professionals
Reduction in fat shaming from the rest of the world

Risks of losing weight for fertility treatment

Decreased quality of life whilst dieting
Disordered eating patterns and increased risk of developing an eating disorder
Weight (plus possibly more) will likely return when you stop dieting
Other physical and mental side effects such as negative effects on your metabolism, depression, stress and increased risk of heart disease to name a few.

The reality that fat people face

To better highlight the inequality that fat people face when seeking fertility treatment, I would like to share, with permission, some anonymous stories that others have shared with me. They will hopefully help you feel less alone in your experience, but you may find them triggering. Please take care of yourself first and foremost and feel free to skip if you cannot read them.

Elizabeth's Story (name changed for identity protection)

I was diagnosed with PCOS at 16 and put on birth control to treat it until I was in my 20's. I developed White Coat Syndrome, and the thought of going to the doctor sent me into a huge episode. I only went when it was absolutely necessary. I stopped taking birth control, and my PCOS symptoms were out of control for about ten years.

I finally went back to my doctor in 2018 due to needing a PAP smear and uncontrolled high blood pressure diagnosed by my eye doctor on a checkup. At that doctor's appointment, we talked about my fertility and if my husband and I wanted to have children. I was already emotional from being at the doctor, so I said yes, and she referred me to a gynaecologist.

I went to see the gynaecologist in a month later and he said because of my age and the PCOS he wanted to refer me to a Fertility Specialist Clinic He prescribed me Metformin in the meantime to help with my PCOS.

During this waiting time to see the specialist, my doctor ordered a number of blood tests to make sure everything was ok with me since it had been so long since I'd had a health check. All my tests came back normal. I also got my period for the first time in a year and finally maybe felt some hope.

Fertility support for fat people

In June, my husband and I went to see the fertility specialist, we felt hopeful, but also fearful as my BMI was very high at the time. When it was our turn to go in for our consult, the first thing the doctor said was, "so you want to get pregnant? Your BMI is over X[5]...that is really harmful", I started to cry controllably as my worst fear just came true. I was fearful he is just going to look at my weight and shame me, and he did. As I said there bawling my eyes out, he continued to state that at my weight and how I was basically going to die in 10 years, and I would never carry a healthy pregnancy. I just cried more. My husband didn't know what to say and didn't say much at the time.

Because I have severe White Coast Syndrome I just froze, thinking over and over to myself I need to leave, this is toxic, but the fear I was going to die just kept coming. The doctor then told me I didn't get a period this past month because I don't ovulate and it's breakthrough bleeding because it lasted more than seven days and prescribed me Prevara to induce a period as he told me I probably had uterine cancer because I don't shed my lining every month. The doctor told me he recommended I get Gastric Bypass Surgery before I went down any road to try and have a baby. Because I was so upset, I just let him sign me up for the program, because if you qualify (which I did, based on my high blood pressure) it's a free surgery and program in Ontario. I left crying uncontrollably, thinking I was going to die, I had cancer, and I would never have a family of my own and completely inconsolable.

Once my husband and I got home, I was finally thinking more clearly, and I got mad. I called MY doctor to make an appointment as soon as I could to tell her what happened at the fertility doctor. My doctor apologized on behalf of that doctor, went over all my bloodwork numbers and reassured me that this doctor didn't know me, my lifestyle or anything about me and just looked at my weight and assumed a lot of wrong things. I went on to get an ultrasound done ordered by my doctor just to check and make sure everything was ok with my ovaries and uterus, and there was nothing, no cysts, no cancer …. NOTHING.

---

[5] Numbers have been substituted to avoid triggering.

My doctor asked me if I wanted to see a dietitian, and the one in their office was great, so I agreed. I saw the dietician at, and I left that appointment feeling amazing.

In a desperate attempt to do something, I started to eat an extremely low carb diet thinking that was the answer. When I dietician saw she explained to me why that wasn't healthy and introduced me to the idea of Intuitive Eating and Health At Every Size, she also looked at my blood work and recommended a bunch of vitamin and supplements to try to help my PCOS.

I am happy to report a year later I haven't lost a pound, but I haven't missed a period since and they are a normal period of 6 days each time like clockwork. I still am on my blood pressure medication, but the medication helps, and I monitor at home, and it's all in a healthy range. My husband went for two sperm analysis, and both came back with low motility, so our fertility issues need a specialist. But due to the trauma I endured from the fertility doctor and talking with another friend of mine who endured the same fat shaming experience at her consultation at another clinic in our region years prior (only difference is she stood up for herself, and she now has twin boys from the results of a successful IUI), and never wanting to do anything too invasive in the first place, my husband and I decided to just keep trying naturally and also pursue adoption for have our family (but that is a whole other story).

I don't give up hope of a miracle happening one day, and I'll have my family naturally, and I know that my body will support it if it does happen, but it took a lot of trauma therapy and self-love to believe that of myself truly.

Anna's Story (name changed for identity protection)

I am a test tube baby I was conceived via IVF in 1998. My mother had the same disease I do, PCOS. This has caused me to have little progesterone and an abnormally high level of testosterone. I have had multiple miscarriages during my young life. I do not necessarily want to have a baby at this moment. I have just come to the realization I may never be able to carry a baby to term. My last miscarriage was November last year.

Gaining all of this information has been a real eye opener for me at even this age. I know the problems I will likely face when I am completely ready to be a parent, and most of those issues will, in doctors opinions, revolve around my weight.

Even though my mom got weight loss surgery after she had me loosing over X lb and she still couldn't conceive, it was not her weight that caused her infertility. And doctors choose to overlook that!

Jasmine's story (name changed for identity protection)

My experience for the past three years has been entirely geared towards me having to lose weight before even attempting to get pregnant.

My doctor constantly tried to force a weight loss drug on me to lose weight. I kept refusing. I have IBS as it is and definitely do not need another medication that makes me literally shit my pants.

When I went to him regarding the fact that I thought I had PCOS, he said no, he doesn't think so. After doing some more research myself, I went back and said I want to be tested for PCOS. His response was "I think you're just looking for an excuse not to lose weight but fine; we'll send you for blood tests."

Of course, my test came back and said my testosterone was off the charts, so he sent me for a scan which confirmed my ovaries had multiple cysts.

Once it was confirmed, nothing more was said. I wasn't offered any support or medication. Again, it was through my own research that I discovered Metformin, and I requested it. I had no advice or information from my doctors about what PCOS meant for me. All I know is what I've learned myself through research and talking to others with it.

Lisa's story (name changed for identity protection)

While my doctor was sympathetic about my fertility issues, they couldn't refer me for anything fertility related. My husband, who has no weight problems, was able to get a couple of sperm tests with no problems. I asked around all the private clinics near me, but as my BMI is/was over 35, they wouldn't treat me. We decided to go to a clinic 2 hours away that was able to help us. Since my only problem is that I don't ovulate naturally, the consultant was astounded that the NHS wouldn't help with something she deemed as very easy to treat. We had a round of IVF, and it was successful, although I, unfortunately, had a missed miscarriage at eight weeks.

Julie's story (name changed for identity protection)

Today marks three years since I had a car crash that changed my life forever. I was five weeks pregnant. The crash caused me to miscarry over the next week following that day.

I've been told by four private doctors who are "not on anyone's side" that I'm so morbidly obese that I "would have miscarried anyway." That is fucking bullshit. What killed my children was a woman who thought her phone was more interesting than looking at the road. I'm hoping that I get the justice I deserve.

Shilpa's story (name changed for identity protection)

I've been through many many cycles of IVF and had two healthy pregnancies. We decided to try for a 3rd baby, and after a few cycles, became pregnant. I'd had a scan at almost seven weeks, and everything looked great, saw a heartbeat etc. we were so excited, but on my way home from the scan I started to bleed and proceeded to have a miscarriage.

I was devastated and returned to my clinic for a follow-up scan to see what was happening a few days later. Sadly they confirmed I had miscarried and wanted me to speak to the doctor after - mine was unavailable so I had to see a female doctor I had never seen before. We sat down in her office, and she looked on screen at my file and my history. She had nothing to say, and the only thing she did say was to tell me that since I'm morbidly obese, I shouldn't be surprised, and that would most likely be the reason why I miscarried. I was devastated and couldn't believe the lack of empathy she had.

It was so wrong to me that moments after confirming I had lost the baby I had been trying so hard for and was so overjoyed about, to be reminded of my weight and for her to assume that was a negative thing and the cause for my situation. I felt sick, but I couldn't escape and had to sit there and listen to this woman make assumptions about me and lecture me, and all I wanted was to break down and cry. It's been three years, and it still effects me. If anything it's given me so much more anxiety around these doctors because she basically said out loud all of the worst most horrible things I always feared these doctors were thinking.

Annette's story (name changed for identity protection)

My husband and I have been trying for three years, and the attitudes of most health professionals has been awful. One of the worst examples was when we were referred to the fertility clinic. The sole focus was on my weight. There wasn't any questions about what my lifestyle is like. The consultant dressed it up as if she was doing me a favour, saying I deserve to lose weight to have a happy and healthy life, and if I wasn't going to lose weight to have a baby then I never would. She started off by saying "you know what I'm going to say, don't you?" I really wish that I'd played ignorant, just to make her feel as awkward as I felt, but instead I went bright red (I don't embarrass easily!) and said "my weight.." My husband tried to jump to my defence - he tried to explain that I do exercise, that I have an eating disorder (I've suffered from bulimia and binge eating disorder on and off for most of my life, thankfully now I'm in recovery) and that I have PCOS which makes losing weight a lot harder, but she wasn't interested at all. She even offered to refer me to Slimming World, even after my husband had told her about my eating disorder.

As soon as we got to the car, I burst into tears. I felt like a failure, and it's put me off going back for any help.

Since then, I've lost around 2 and a half stone, and ironically it's since I've stopped caring about how I look and instead focus on eating intuitively and exercising to feel good. I'm still overweight, and recently saw my GP who asked if I want referred to the fertility clinic (my husband and I have relocated to a different area so it would be a different clinic) and I told her my concerns. She said I should try and lose weight, and whilst she wasn't as pushy about it as others have been, she certainly didn't say "your weight doesn't matter."

What frustrates me the most is I'm 5"2, and because the NHS are strict about BMI, I've been told for my height I'd need to be between X and a half stone - X and a half stone to be the ideal weight. I can't remember being that weight! Even when I was thin (my weight has always fluctuated), I was a UK size X/X, and had hips and a chubby tummy.

I just wish that to access fertility help, clinics and professionals would take an holistic approach rather than taking a look at a woman in a fat body and determine whether she deserves help or not.

Chapter 3 - My quest for thinness

I can't remember a time when I wasn't conscious of my weight. Looking back at photos of me as a child, I looked like any other kid. Wading through photo albums, I really can't see at what point I started worrying about the way I looked. My first memory of being picked on for being fat was name-calling in the playground when I was about 8. I don't remember the specifics, just that feeling of not being like the other kids, singled out for being different. I can remember that awkward feeling inside of not being sure why I was different or what I could do about it.

I still remember vividly when food first became a "thing" for me. It all started with my after-school snacks. My sister and I went to our grandparents after school when my parents were at work, and they always had these delicious crisps in their cupboard. Even now, I can remember the pure pleasure I got from eating them. At some point when I was at primary school, my beloved crisps were swapped for a lower calorie option. I know that the intention behind this decision was from a place of love, but for me, that was the start of seeing food as good and bad. My sister still ate the crisps that I loved, but because of the way that my body was, that meant that I didn't deserve to eat the food that I liked so much.

These smalls changes in my diet eventually led to attending weight loss classes. My mum and I must have tried them all in an attempt to lose weight. "Dancing in the Moonlight" by Toploader (a great 90s classic pop song) was forever ruined for me by a dancing routine at a weight loss group.

Whether it was calories or points, picking a green day or a red day (WTF?), I remember food taking over my life. If I wasn't eating, I was thinking about what

I was going to eat or what I couldn't eat. If I'd eaten something "off plan" then I was beating myself up mentally and trying to figure out how I could a) hide it b) counteract it with exercise or c) avoid eating later to make up for it.

Thinking about food was relentless. My mood was entirely dependent upon the number on the scale every morning, and on what sized clothes I could fit into. My confidence in my body was in shatters. I went to an all girl's high school, which on the whole, I loved. I started out there as a pretty confident, smart young woman. I was good at public speaking. I was generally a good student and made some great friends there.

It did nothing to help my confidence around boys, though. I can remember the first time a boy asked me out as if it was yesterday (which is pretty impressive considering I can't remember what happened yesterday!) Most days after school, all the kids from the local high schools would flock into the city centre (and when I say city, don't get impressed, it's tiny!) and hang out by the fountain or on the hall steps. This is where the cool kids hung out. One day, one boy (a friend of a friend I think) came over to me and asked me out (or some other lame phrase - this was pre-social media, and we'd only just got mobile phones, so social interaction was an entirely different ball game) This poor boy though, getting up the courage to ask out a girl he liked. The thing I remember most is my reaction. I laughed in his face. I couldn't stop myself. Not because he wasn't a nice looking lad, not because I thought he was an idiot, but because I thought it was so ridiculous that anyone would want to ask me out, that anyone would think that I was pretty or worth spending more time with. This wasn't a pity party, or a "woe is me" response. This was a genuine "oh my god you can't be serious" fit of hysterics. I honestly thought he was making fun of me.

Looking back at that now makes me so sad. That poor young woman who couldn't even believe that someone would find her attractive. That it was so absurd to her that someone would choose her, that she laughed in his face. I really wish I could go back and give her a big hug and tell her just how worthy she is of being loved. What makes me even sadder is that I had loving parents and good friends. My life was peachy on the outside, so I cannot even begin to imagine how hard it is for others whose lives weren't as privileged as mine.

It was at 16 that I was diagnosed with Polycystic Ovary Syndrome (PCOS). PCOS is a group of symptoms they lump together to explain a set of hormonal and metabolic changes. It's poorly understood even now and back then (a good 20 years ago) it was even less understood. When the doctor diagnosed me, she immediately followed up her diagnosis with the bombshell that I wouldn't be able to have kids. I had no idea then, but looking back now, it had a significant impact on my mental health. My grades at 16 were fantastic but then things started to slide, my A level results were good but not as good as they should have been and then at university I left with a "drinkers" degree of a 2:2. Somehow I still managed to get into a prestigious masters degree (I don't think they knew how to turn me away once they'd offered me a place) but I knew that I wasn't fulfilling my potential and I knew my health and my serious self-confidence issues were the reason why.

Luckily the doctor was wrong (more on this later), and I was able to have my two boys with ease, but it wasn't by losing weight or "curing" my PCOS. In fact, I was classed as high-risk during both my pregnancies due to my weight. And even after I'd had my children, I still wasn't happy with my body.

The big realisation

After I'd had my babies, I half-heartedly tried a few other restrictive eating plans in the guise of eating healthily. I ate no sugar for six weeks - and promptly fell off the so-called wagon the following day. I tried intermittent fasting for a few months, but you know what, I was so fed up. I was already bloody exhausted from learning how to be a mum, the endless sleepless nights, and I just did not have the energy to put myself through dieting. I wanted to enjoy spending time with my kids, I didn't want to spend my time thinking about food, and I did not have the mental energy.

Nicola Salmon

I looked back at my life, and all I saw was my years defined by which diet I was following at the time and what dress size I was. No matter what size I was (which varied hugely from size 12 to size 24), I was never happy, and I always saw myself as fat. The realisation smacked me in the face. My happiness did not depend on my size. If it did, I would have been much happier at the size 12 than at the size 24, but it didn't make a difference. I felt exactly the same, unhappy and unworthy. So if my happiness didn't depend on my weight, then what the hell was I doing with my life? Why was I wasting all my mental energy worrying about this shit every single day? What was the point? I wasn't getting thinner or healthier; I was getting fatter and more depressed.

I was sat waiting for a train one day about a year ago, and I found an old note on my phone. I'd written it four years earlier when I was on (another) diet. It was an exercise they got you to do right at the beginning of the diet to motivate you into losing weight, a list of all the things I could do when I lost weight.

This is what my list looked like:
- Wear skinny jeans tucked into knee-high boots
- Buy jeans that fit perfectly
- Go on a swing
- Wear a bikini

I saw this list and almost said out loud "what the actual fuck!" I don't need to wait to do all these things? Who the hell said I can't wear skinny jeans tucked into knee-high boots right now? Why the hell were these things only ok when I was a certain weight? What was I worried about? That I was going to be so heavy for the swing that I was going to break the swing and die of embarrassment? Maybe, but come on, why I am so worried about what other people think, that I'm not actually living my life?

51

The pact

So that's when I made a pact with myself. I was not going to go on another diet, and I was never going to weigh myself ever again. Why?

The restrictive nature of dieting took over my whole life. I lived and breathed dieting. But that is not what I wanted for my life anymore. I didn't want to be obsessed with food, for it to take up my every waking moment and stress me out. I've got bigger stuff to do with my life than worry about that. And although I do still think about food, I probably think about it a quarter of the amount of time I used to now, compared with a few years ago. I don't beat myself up about eating a doughnut, maybe when I eat five but it's a journey, right?

The no scales thing has probably been even harder to give up. That number of the scale defined me. If it was going down, I was a good girl, and it made me feel good about myself but if it was going up or staying the same that meant I was awful and needed to beat myself up a bit more so that I could motivate myself to lose weight again.

After being defined by this number my whole life, when I gave it up, suddenly I had to find a new way to define myself. There was space to choose who I wanted to be. At the moment I'm choosing to put all my energy and passion into my business, maybe not the healthiest choice, but it's giving me an identity where I could get so easily lost in being "just" a mum. Right now, writing this book and working with fat women who want to start their families feels so much more important than losing weight.

If you could choose (and you can) how would you define yourself? If you could smash up the scales, cut out all the labels in your clothes, and forget all those infertility "labels" you've been given, how would you want to define who you are?

You are more than just a number. You are capable of incredible things. You get to choose what those things are and use your precious time and energy to do them. Don't waste your energy worrying about that number and what other people think about that number. Chances are there are so concerned about their own number that they don't even notice yours.

So you have a choice today. You have a choice every day. Are you going to be defined by that number on the scale or the labels you've attached to yourself? Or are you going to skip the weigh in today and instead choose to define yourself by your kick-ass achievements, your incredible goals or just the fact that right now you are inherently worthy of everything you want regardless of anything - your weight, your past, your job, your health, your decisions, your mental health, anything.

When weight loss is taken off the table, so many of my clients start taking steps to goals that really matter to them. They start taking better care of their bodies, feeling better in their daily lives and most importantly living their life, instead of putting it on hold for a time when they have lost weight.

Chapter 4 - The FAT+ve fertility framework

If weight loss isn't the problem and diets don't work, what the hell can we do now? How can you support your body to getting pregnant without resorting to the one thing you've known all your life?

Instead of focusing on the arbitrary number on the scale, why not instead focus on want you want to achieve, discovering what things boost your energy or finding a tangible way to measure your fitness? The goal of getting pregnant is so important, but it an impossible goal to work towards. You are either pregnant, or you're not. There is no middle ground to work with; you cannot slowly improve and see the benefits of things shifting. So instead of focusing on getting pregnant right now, we are going to focus on other, more tangible goals that are going to get you a step closer.

I'm sure weight-tracking has been your method of choice for all if not most health endeavours over the years. For me, it's been the one constant. Anytime I've done something to change my health, it's always been to lose weight, and I have always tracked it by weighing myself on the scales, sometimes daily, sometimes weekly but always regularly. Like if I didn't weigh myself for a while that my weight would somehow explode.

It got to a point where I was addicted to weighing myself. It wasn't even about the actual number in the end, but I had to weigh myself and keep myself in check. What the scale said made a massive difference to my mood. I always had an expectation of how much I'd "deserved" to lose that week, based on what I'd given up, how much I'd deprived myself and how much I'd tortured myself through exercise. But more often than not, I'd be disappointed. Even if I had lost weight, it wouldn't be as much as I'd hoped. There were very few occasions I was ever happy when I got off the scales.

Tracking your weight quickly becomes an addiction and something that's very hard to give up. But this is something I'd strongly encourage you to do. Why? Because it's a meaningless number that sets you up to fail every time. There is absolutely no benefit to weighing yourself. You can argue with me all you want about using it to track your progress as you get healthier, BUT there are far more valuable indicators of health, that will encourage you to live your life healthier and happier instead of finding the next quick fix to lose a few more pounds. If you're anything like me and have been tracking your weight for a long time then giving it up can feel like giving up a friend (all be it a bitchy friend who always tells you your bum looks big)

It's crucial not to go cold turkey and instead replace the weighing for an alternative focus for your health. By switching your attention, you won't mourn the loss of those scales in the same way. If you are willing to go all in, I definitely recommend finding your biggest hammer and smashing those scales to pieces. It's more than just getting rid of your scales; it's a symbolic act that these scales no longer control you and define who you are. You are free. I smashed my glass scales to smithereens (and I'm still finding the pieces in my back garden!)

The Fat-Positive Framework

While working with women in fat bodies who want to get pregnant, I realised that we face unique challenges. We can't just go to our doctor and ask for the support that we need (although one day I hope that will be the case!). With our current medical system, so many women face judgement and shame for being in a bigger body.

The FAT +ve fertility framework

I created the FAT+ve framework to give us the tools we need to get pregnant in our fat bodies.

F- Formulate: Create an action plan that does not centre around weight loss but takes you from where you are right now to your health goals and priorities in a way that feels good.

A- Advocate: Arm yourself with the tools to advocate for your body with other healthcare professionals. Learn how to ask for the support that you deserve and demand better from your doctor.

T - Trust: Relearn how to trust your body in a world where we are told to ignore what our body is telling us. We are so used to using external cues that we have forgotten how to listen to what our body needs.

+ve - Positive: When you have been told that you can't get pregnant because you are too fat, it's essential to retrain your brain into believing that your body is capable of getting pregnant

Once you've gotten rid of the scales, use the first step in the framework, **Formulate**, to begin to focus on your needs and priorities when it comes to your health.

Here are some ideas of other ways to start tracking your health. Pick one that makes the most sense for you and try using it in place of the scales.

Pick your favourite movement/exercise and find a way to measure it so you can see your improvement. e.g. you can walk/run/cycle the same route a bit faster; you can swim more lengths without taking a break, you can lift heavier weights at the gym, you can stretch further in your yoga poses.

Use a habit tracker to track your consistency with your healthy habits like drinking enough water, eating foods that make you feel good, meditation, taking your vitamins, etc.

Pick an area of health that you want to improve and track it. e.g. maybe you need more sleep, you'd like your cycle to be more regular, or you want to reduce your IBS symptoms.

Think about what would be the best indicator for your health and go with it. Be curious and explore what works best for your body.

If you want an all in one health tracker, grab a copy of The Nurture Fertility Journal, where you can track your Basal Body Temperature (BBT), your habits, your daily nutrition, movement, water intake, energy, mood, sleep and more.

Exercise

I'm going to walk you through my favourite exercise to formulate your own plan, not based on how many pounds or kilos you can lose but based on your needs and priorities for your own health.

You can download a sheet to follow along with inside the "Fat and Fertile" accompanying PDF that contains all the exercises from the book that you can fill in straight on your computer or print off. Access the PDF at nicolasalmon.co.uk/bookbonus

Step One
Your first step is to write down how you feel about different areas of your life right now on a scale of 0 - 10. 0 is the lowest you can imagine. 10 is your ideal life where everything is just as you want it. Rate each section:
Physical health: How you feel in your body.

Emotional health: How you feel emotionally.
Relationships: Any meaningful relationships in your life.
Lifestyle: How you spend your time and balance your life.
Financial health: How you feel about your finances
Spiritual health

Step Two
For each segment, write down 2-5 things that you'd like to do, be or how that would make that area of your life 10 out of 10.

Step Three
Now I'd like you to pick 1-2 areas which are the most important for you and which would make the most significant difference to your quality of life right now.

Step Four
Based on these 1-2 priorities and thinking about the next week only, what tiny steps can you do to move you closer to your 10 out of 10 life. Write down 1-5 actions that you can commit to for this week.

Once you have those steps written down, I want you to check in with yourself.

Are these steps manageable for this week?
Are these steps small enough?
What things might get in the way this week?
How can I ensure I will be successful?
How can I make it easy for myself?

At the end of your week, come back and reflect on how your week went.

> What went well?
> Did anything get in your way?
> Looking at your priorities, what steps next week are going to have the biggest impact?

Thin doesn't not equal fertile.

When you are fat, you imagine that being thin will solve all your problems, I certainly did.

"When I'm thin, I'll have more friends; my business will be more successful, I'll have more money, I'll be invited to so many amazing places.........................."

We seem to think that being thin is going to fix everything. But it doesn't. Thin does not equal fertile. If you severely restrict the calories available to your body or do extreme exercise, your body will shut down your periods completely (this condition is known as hypothalamic amenorrhea).

In the caveman days, this was a great advantage, evolutionary speaking. It meant that when food was in short supply or you were in danger from predators frequently, your body wouldn't have to lose valuable resources on your period or deal with being pregnant. The extra resources that it needs to be pregnant may have caused you to starve or get killed, so your body shuts it down altogether. Makes sense, right?

Your body doesn't know the difference between the cabbage soup diet and a lack of food to eat in a drought. It doesn't know that you're intentionally trying to lose weight to try and get pregnant. It's just trying to keep you safe. That's all your body ever wants to do. Your body does not hate you.

The idea that your body is working against you can make life hard. When you feel like you need to fight against your body, you are putting all your energy into working against what your body needs to do. Your body is infinitely more intelligent than our brains. It does a million different things each second without us even having to think about it. Right now, it is doing the very best it can to function optimally in the environment it is in. You don't blame the flower for not growing. Instead, you change the soil, give it more water, put it in the sun. You make changes so that the flow can flourish. How can you make small changes so that you and your body can flourish? What are you letting your body get in the way of?

Sometimes my body gets in the way of things I want to do, but it's not the fat's fault. More often than not (and nearly every example I can think of except certain yoga positions), it's actually my thoughts about my fat body getting in my way. My perception of what my body is capable of and what other people would think of me gets in the way much more often.

Chapter 5 - How to advocate for your fat body

The second area of the FAT+ve fertility framework is A for **Advocate**. As we live in a world that isn't designed for fat bodies, we need to be able to advocate for ourselves and our bodies in order to have our rights, and our needs met.

This can be from your doctor and healthcare team, but you also might need to advocate for yourself with your friends and family and even strangers, When it comes to fat bodies, everyone feels like they can have an opinion, and they often feel the need to express it "for your health!"

Fat Shaming

If you are living in a fat body, you are well aware that fat shaming is a very real type of bullying in this day and age. Grown adults think it's entirely acceptable for comment and shame you for how your body looks on a daily basis and this behaviour is positively encouraged everywhere we go.

No matter what you go to see your doctor about, it's likely she will mention your weight as the problem. Recently a campaign has been launched by Cancer Research UK (who funnily enough receive huge donations from Slimming World) that is everywhere. The campaign states that the second biggest cause of cancer after smoking is ….. obesity. The research behind this is dubious at best, and the results are damaging. This campaign will not encourage more people to lose weight. What it will do is further stigmatise those of us in bigger bodies and segregate us further from society.

How to advocate for your fat body

In a dystopian future (think "The Handmaids Tale" by Margaret Atwood) I can see people with fat bodies being forced to pay more for our healthcare because we are fat. We will be denied more and more healthcare options based on our size; we will pay more health insurance because we are deemed higher risk, our decisions about our own health will be further and further reduced. To be honest, this isn't so far from the truth right now. I already pay more for my life insurance than my husband based on my BMI.

When I had my first son, I was classified morbidly obese on the BMI scale. This meant that I was deemed a high-risk pregnancy, even though there was no evidence that I was in any kind of ill health. I had a very healthy pregnancy. When I was making my choice around our birth, I wanted a water birth at home. I had done my research, and this was my choice. This was how I wanted to bring my son into the world. The problem was I was too fat. I had to fight very hard for this idea to be even entertained. They kept bringing up these "significant risks" that could happen (shoulder dystocia, being too heavy to move in an emergency) all of which were not backed up by research. I was discouraged and made to feel completely irresponsible every step of the way.

In the end, I had the birth I didn't want, and I was coerced into agreeing to things that, when in labour, I wasn't in any state to agree to. Birth was not the empowering experience I had wanted and the reason? I was too fat. I was dangerous. All through this process, I felt like I was putting my son at risk. Not because I was (I researched my decisions thoroughly and knew the risks and benefits of each of my decisions) but because everyone around me was telling me I was wrong and that because I had a fat body, I couldn't do all the things I wanted to do.

How do you feel about getting pregnant whilst you're fat? What have people told you about this? I'd bet large sums of money that at least one person has commented on your fat and how detrimental it will be to pregnancy, birth and motherhood. Everyone feels like they have an opinion on this!

Nicola Salmon

Do you feel unworthy of becoming a mother?

Do you feel that because of your fat body, you are an awful person and that you do not deserve to get pregnant? Where does this come from? It's a horrid thought, isn't it? You would never in a million years say this to anyone else, yet you think it to yourself (maybe only subconsciously) every day. If you don't believe you deserve to get pregnant, what impact do you think that's going to have on your ability to get pregnant?

Let's look at the evidence.

What does having a fat body really mean about you? It means you have fat cells on your body. That's it. Those fat cells do not directly affect your behaviour. It does not make you mean, or unkind, or greedy, or stupid, or ugly or anything else. Your associations, previous experiences and beliefs give the fat that meaning.

This is what a fat body means to me (Go with me on this!) You have fat cells on your body, right? Fat is purely stored energy. Energy you are saving for later. Scientifically, Power is energy converted over time. I like to think that the fat cells around my body are my unexpressed power. All those times that you felt that you couldn't speak up. That your power was taken away from you, you didn't lose that power. That power is still available to you. You've stored it away for later, but it still belongs to you.

That beautiful belly, those powerful thighs contain your power. Think of the things that you can do with that power and energy? The things that you can achieve, the ways you can stand up for yourself and speak out. You are a powerful woman. You are capable of incredible things. You may have been told otherwise your whole life. You may have been told to take up less and less space. You've probably been told that you need to shrink yourself to be a good girl.

How to advocate for your fat body

It's ok to take up space. Take up more space. Demand equal rights that are given to others in smaller bodies. Speak up when you are discriminated against. Use your power!

Worthiness is another one of these beliefs. You choose what you are worthy of, whether you are doing it consciously or unconsciously. Not only are you inherently worthy of being a mother - I believe every woman is if that is what she wants. You are also worthy of love and most importantly, self-love.

What does that mean? It means that you are worthy of taking care of yourself. You are worthy of making sure you eat foods that are going to make you feel good in your body. You are worthy of spending your free time doing things that make you fill up with joy. You are worthy of making little decisions every day that nourish your physical and mental health, not deplete you.

Our worth as women in the society we live is not appreciated. In fact, we are so undervalued that women still only get paid 85% of what men get paid for the same job. (This statistic was from 2018). We are supposed to be good girls, seen but not heard, smiling and looking nice for the benefit of men. For the thousands of years in which we have lived in a patriarchal society, that has been our role, that has been our worth. But that is not our real worth.

When we stand up and claim our rights as equal humans in our society, we reclaim our worth as humans who can look exactly as they choose to - fat and all! Whose sole purpose in life isn't to please other people but to please ourselves. So how are you taking care of yourself? In your day to day life, what decisions are you basing on your worth? The food you choose? How you travel? The things you buy? The clothes you wear?

How do you make these decisions? And where does your perceived worth come into this? Being able to make choices in these areas is a very privileged position to be it.

Clothes are a huge area of this for me. For the longest time, I only bought cheap, ill-fitting clothes. My "logical" reasoning for this was that I was going to lose weight so I wouldn't be wearing them for very long. What was the point in spending lots of money on clothes that I wasn't going to be wearing for a long time? Do you know what my subconscious was saying? You are not worthy of nice clothes. You are fat, ugly and not worthy of clothes that fit well. Why waste money on beautiful clothes just to put them on your fat, ugly body?

For the longest time, I was stuck in a downward spiral. I didn't feel worthy in my body. I felt like my body meant that I wasn't able to wear certain clothes (basically anything I liked!) eat to certain places (because I always felt like I stood out) and trying new things because I was worried that people would laugh at me. Haha, look at that fat girl trying to rock climb - as if!

My adventurous streak has been hidden away for a long time because I couldn't bear to be humiliated, and this unworthiness seeped into my everyday decisions, especially how I took care of myself. The self is a tough thing to define. The outward appearance of you is your body, but you are so much more than just your body. The fact that you even call it your body rather than just you, points to a much larger picture.

But when it came to taking care of myself, my body and the larger picture took a hit. I punished it all. I didn't feel worthy enough to eat food I really enjoyed, so I ate food that made me feel rubbish, I didn't feel worthy of moving my body in ways that I enjoyed so I either tortured myself with exercise I hated or did nothing. I didn't take care of my body in any way really, and that made me hate it even more. I'm sure I could list at least a hundred different ways that I didn't like my body. But who was this really serving?

My body is the only one I've got, so why am I so bloody unkind to it? Why do I not deserve to eat food that makes me feel good? Why am I not allowed to move my body in ways that feel good? Why can't I use body products to look after my body and make myself feel good? Just because my body is fat does not mean that it is unworthy of love and taking care of in the best possible way. All this was an example of how I had internalised the fat phobia around me.

It's not just other people who can fat shame us. We can (and do!) fat shame ourselves every minute of every day. We have been surrounded by messages that tell us fat is unhealthy for so long that we need to unlearn all those ways in which it has filtered into our everyday thoughts.

One of the easiest ways we can start to unpick our own internal fat-phobia is to stop commenting on other people's bodies. Commenting on other's bodies and clothes is a socially acceptable thing to do, but whether you are saying (or thinking) positive or negative things about someone, you are judging them based on how their body looks. Try to focus on other things about a person and not comment at all on their body. We need to allow all bodies to be just as they are. Not criticised or judged. And we need to remove the hate we direct towards our own bellies, they are the environment we want to grow our babies in.

What about what others think?

So maybe you can get on board with learning to respect your fat body, after all, it does some pretty phenomenal things. But what about everyone else? Everyone has an opinion about your health if you're fat and if you tell them you're trying to get pregnant. The combination makes you easy prey.

What can you do about everyone else's fat-phobic remarks, rude comments and unsolicited advice? My advice to you is to fuck em all! You cannot change other people, so there is no point in wasting your energy. Save your energy for you.

If it is someone close to you who is causing you a problem, you can explain to them exactly how hurtful their comments are and that you will not tolerate them anymore. There need to be some big boundaries, and you need to stand firm with them. They are essential for your mental health. If people are constantly wearing you down with their "well-meaning" advice, it will be challenging to continue to respect this awesome body you have. If they persist with their comments, avoid. Don't worry about hurting their feelings. You need to protect you right now. Unfollow them on social media. Don't reply to their messages and avoid them if you can.

These boundaries need to extend to all areas of your life, and as a generation, we do spend a lot of time online, so do a social media cull. Block and delete anyone who triggers you when you see their posts. Don't worry, it doesn't have to be forever, but it's essential that you surround yourself with positivity in what you see right now.

If you need some inspiration here are just a small handful of amazing people on Instagram, you can check out and follow:

@fatpositivefertility (me!) @bodyposipanda @lottielamour @katstroudofficial @sofiehagendk @haes_studentdoctor @scarrednotscared @meg.boggs @plusmommy @nerdabouttown @foodpeacedietitian @a_body_well_fed @fyeahmfabello @satisfynutrition @tastingabundance @iamdaniadriana @bodyimage_therapist

How to make empowered health decisions

I'm sure you've been to the doctor with an issue (maybe related to fertility, maybe not) and had the doctor insist that your weight is the issue - regardless of what the issue is. I've had my weight used as a cause of depression, infections, thrush, basically anything I've been to see the doctor about since I was 15.

Having free healthcare in the UK means that it's easy to take a pill for every ailment. If something is wrong, you go to the doctor; they tell you what's wrong, you take a pill and get better. The problem with this type of system is that it completely takes the power away from you as the patient. You are told what is wrong and told what to do. Now I'm not saying that we don't need doctors. Doctors are an essential (and under-appreciated) resource of the system but historically have wielded complete power. There was no room for the patient to make any decision about their own health, especially women (but that's a whole other book).

Things are changing, but we need to embrace that change ourselves. It's up to you to get your voice heard. It's up to you to ask what the options are, what the alternative is, what the risks and benefits are, what the research is. It's your body, and you get to decide what happens to it.

It wasn't until I got pregnant that I was in a situation where I felt strongly enough to advocate for my own health. Before that, I just went along with what I was told, believing that my doctor always knew what was best for me. We live in unprecedented times, where we have access to all the same resources and research as any doctor. Information is power and whilst you may not have done a seven year medical degree, that shouldn't stop you from informing yourself on things that affect you. Your own lived experience with any health condition is valuable and relevant and should not be dismissed.

As with anything, it's a balance between giving yourself the power to make an informed choice and spending all your time on google endlessly researching everything. It can become all-consuming and the problem with the internet is that anyone can put anything up there and often will. So as well as being informed about the information out there, you also have to be discerning about what information to put value on and what information you take with a pinch of salt.

When I first began to advocate for my own health, I suddenly realised how thousands of years of oppression of women's bodies were still interweaved into healthcare. I read stories of doctors giving women extra stitches when sewing up their vaginas after birth without their consent to tighten things up for their husband's pleasure. I experienced first hand when giving birth that my choices and decisions were not listened to. This has been happening to women for thousands of years and even more so for women of colour. There are substantial racial differences in outcomes of different healthcare problems. One that was highlighted recently by Serena Williams, the famous tennis player, was the difference in maternal motility rates between black, non-white and white women.

So how do you make empowered decisions around your own healthcare?

The first step is actually to understand that you can. That you are able to make these decisions yourself. Your doctor gives you advice. That is it. It is their opinion based on their clinical experience. It is your choice how you use this advice. Once you understand that you do have a say in your own health and wellbeing, then it's your chance to speak out.

The next step is to engage. Talk to your doctor about what options you have available. What alternative medications there are. What lifestyle changes you can make. What alternative treatments have research to support them (think acupuncture, physiotherapy, herbal medicine etc.) What would happen if you did nothing? What are the risks of each treatment?

How to advocate for your fat body

Without all this knowledge, you cannot make the best decision for you. If your doctor isn't able to provide this information, you can find it yourself. Research what medications there are out there, look at the side effects. Check the medication package insert. It should be inside any medicines you have and can be found online. It gives you the common side effects of any medication. Speak to other healthcare practitioners that support fertility to find out what else could benefit you.

The final step is to listen to your gut. Sure there may be a logical choice when you are making the decision about your healthcare, but sometimes you will have a strong sense of what the right thing is for you. This is your intuition calling. Don't ignore it. Sometimes it might not be the logical choice, but it's the right choice for you. Follow your gut and decide what the right thing for you now is.

You know what? You can change your mind. Keep asking questions, keep weighing the risks vs the benefits, and if you decide to change what you want to do, that's ok. You don't have to explain yourself to anyone. You don't have to feel bad for changing your mind or inconveniencing people.

So how might this play out in real life?

A great example is IVF. There are so many choices to make, especially if you are paying for your own treatment. You can choose which clinic you go to, which consultant you see, what testing you have beforehand, what protocol you use, which drugs, what quantities of each drug, how many embryos to put back, the list goes on. Your doctor will advise you which things make the most sense based on your previous health history but if you have a sense that there is something additional you want testing or that you would prefer to try a different drug (especially if you previously experience an adverse reaction with a particular drug before) then don't be afraid to discuss these things with your doctor.

Say you suffer from IBS - a common stress-related digestive complaint that can often be linked with high levels of inflammation. You've read information about immune factors playing a role in fertility and would like to take this further. You mention it to your doctor, but he tells you its not relevant.

What can you do? You have choices! You have options! Talk to your doctor again. Explain why you feel it's an issue and what course you would like to take. Ask them for research around their opinion (especially if they dismiss you out of hand) and for all the options and risk vs benefits for each option you could take.

If you are not satisfied with your doctor, ask for a second opinion - either someone at the clinic, you are already at or at a different clinic. Even if it's just a preliminary chat to find out more about their services, remember at the end of the day, they are providing you with a service (no matter how much you are paying out of pocket - you are paying for this one way or another) and as the customer, you should be completely satisfied with the service they are giving you. If you're still not satisfied - research more about the condition and relevant clinics that might be able to help you. Listen to your gut and find the answer that you need.

Word of warning: Fertility research can become obsessive. There is so much information online, and most of it is based on little if any evidence. Take note of where the information is coming from and be sensible about the risks you take with your health.

A really common example that I see time and time again is fat women being turned away from their doctors without any support. The conversation usually goes something like this:

You: "My husband and I have been trying to get pregnant for the last 18 months, but nothing is happening. What can we do?"

Doctor: "Do you have regular cycles?"

You: "My cycles are normally regular but can sometimes be a bit erratic."

Doctor: "How much do you weight?"

You: "mumble mumble, I'm not really sure."

Doctor: "Let's get you on the scales..........ok so using the BMI scale you are clinically obese. If you want to get pregnant, you need to lose weight."

You: "I eat healthily, and I exercise a couple of times a week, what more can I do?"

Doctor: "Hmm, maybe try a more restrictive diet? Come back in 3 months when you've lost some weight, and we'll see what we can do."

What is wrong with this conversation? The doctor is assuming that you are living an unhealthy lifestyle without really going into much detail. They aren't offering you any support around nutrition or movement. They've given you no idea of what might be going on with your fertility, only that they think your weight is a factor. What could you do differently?

You can question the assumptions that the doctor is making about your health. Reiterate to the doctor that you do have a healthy lifestyle and your diet is not contributing to your weight issues. Ask to see the evidence for that weight loss improves fertility. The doctor's job is to base his clinical decisions on evidence-based medicine to ensure that this is what they are doing. Decide what course of action you want before you go in and fight for this. Maybe you want to have your hormones checked with a blood test. If you know what you want going in and what benefit that will have for you, you are much more likely to request it and get it.

Ask questions. The more questions you ask, the more informed you'll be about the decisions around your health. Ask what the alternatives are. Ask why things should be a certain way. Ask what the benefits and risks are. Ask them what their course of action would be for a patient in a smaller body and then ask for that.

If the doctor refuses a particular treatment or test, ask them to document that on your medical record. This can sometimes push them to agree to your requested outcome. If your doctor isn't giving you satisfactory answers, exercise your right to see another doctor. Your doctor is there to provide you with a service, ensure you are getting the service that you deserve.

Boundaries can be another constructive way to frame your conversation with your doctor. Go into your appointment being really clear about what your boundaries are. What is and isn't ok for you. You are entirely within your rights to ask not to be weighed and for certain topics such as weight loss and diet/lifestyle changes to be off the table.

Ragen Chastain wrote an empowering blog post "What to Say at the Doctor's Office".[6] In her article she highlighted the weight bias she has received and shared her wisdom about how to advocate for yourself if you are in a position to do so.

She writes, "Over the years I've developed some strategies that help me deal with health care professionals who are harboring weight bias. By far the one I use most often when I'm told that something is caused by my weight is "Do thin people get [this issue]." The answer is always yes so I follow up with "What do you prescribe to them? Let's try that." I also talk about research, including asking the doctor how, when there isn't a single study where more than a tiny fraction of people lost weight, and no study that shows they were healthier for it, does she think weight loss qualifies as evidence-based medicine?"

---

[6] https://danceswithfat.org/2013/04/01/what-to-say-at-the-doctors-office/

In the blog post, she also includes a useful card containing helpful phrases you can print out and take with you to your doctor. These phrases include:

"Show me a study where a majority of subjects succeeded at the amount of weight loss you are suggesting.

Do thin people get this health problem? What do you recommend for them?

Please provide me with evidence based medicine and the opportunity for informed consent"

The research

It can be helpful to bring in some research that supports your arguments when you go and see your healthcare team. Below is a summary of some of the current research alongside the references. You can find a printable copy of this in the "Fat to Fertile" PDF so that you can take it with you to your doctors. Access the PDF at nicolasalmon.co.uk/bookbonus

Trigger warning - the majority of the research still contains fat-phobic language and ideas.

Amongst the large set of research data that shows a correlation between BMI and fertility issues, and draws the conclusion that being in a bigger body means that it is irresponsible to get pregnant, are some thought-provoking articles that address the inequality and discrimination faced by people in bigger bodies who need support getting pregnant.

In 2010 S. Pandey et al. wrote a debate brief for Human Reproduction looking at the arguments for denying access to fertility treatment based on BMI.[7] They concluded that all the arguments used for excluding women based on their BMI had a poor quality of evidence to back them up.

For the argument that IVF and other ART had poor success for women with higher BMI, Pandey stated that "A systemic review on the effect of overweight and obesity in women undergoing assisted reproductive techniques concluded that there was insufficient evidence to link high BMI with reduced birth rates".

For the argument that people with higher BMI have increased risks on obstetric and perinatal complications, Pandey argues that although he sees an increase in risk with BMI, clinicians do not take into account the negative impact of age when asking patients to lose weight and that "the upper limit of BMI compatible with an acceptable risk profile in pregnancy is still to be determined"

Cost is also considered and Pandey shows that "a recent study failed to show any significant differences in cost per live birth following ART in overweight and obese women"

Pandey also highlights that many BMI cut off values are arbitrary and not based on any evidence. They also discuss the poor success associated with interventions for weight loss and that "the impact of most dietary interventions is short lived and weight lost is often regained over time"

In 2017, Koning et al. also published a debate entitled "It is not justified to reject fertility treatment based on obesity" in Human Reproduction, looking at

---

[7] Pandey, S. et al., 2010. Should access to fertility treatment be determined by female body mass index?. *Human Reproduction*, [Online]. Volume 25, Issue 4,, 815–820. Available at: https://academic.oup.com/humrep/article/25/4/815/700269 [Accessed 5 February 2019].

the arguments based on risks for women, risks for the future child and importance for society.[8]

When discussing risks for the woman, Koning et al. highlight that there are no additional risks for women when undergoing IVF, but there are higher risks associated with pregnancy complications. They argue that, although the risk is higher, "it does not mean that it is irresponsible to take that risk" and that "a competent and well-informed woman, in principle, has the right to her own deliberation when considering risk taken for herself".

With regards to the risks for the future child, Koning states that in the Netherlands a stance has been formed that "the rejection of treatment on the grounds of the welfare of the child can only be considered in exceptional circumstances, actually when there is 'great risk of serious harm' to the child.

With regards to consequences for society, Koning argues that although costs were higher when looking at pregnancy complications, "excluding women with other comorbidities is not called for."

In an article entitled "Irresponsibly Infertile? Obesity, Efficiency and Exclusion from Treatment" published in Health Care Analysis,[9] Brown goes into great detail to look at the possible justifications for denying people with a higher BMI fertility treatment.

---

[8]Koning, A. et al., 2017. It is not justified to reject fertility treatment based on obesity. *Human Reproduction Open*, [Online]. Volume 2017, Issue 2, hox009. Available at: https://academic.oup.com/hropen/article/2017/2/hox009/4049574 [Accessed 3 February 2019].

[9] Brown, R., 2019. Irresponsibly Infertile? Obesity, Efficiency, and Exclusion from Treatment. *Health Care Analysis*, [Online]. Volume 27, Issue 2, 61–76. Available at: https://link.springer.com/article/10.1007/s10728-019-00366-w [Accessed 29 May 2019].

The first proposition, that "IVF is Futile of Obese Women" Brown states that "it seems unlikely to be appropriate to describe IVF treatments as futile in obese women" due to the fact that "analysis of a large sample of cycles in North America showed live birth artesian morbidly obese women (those with a BMI over 35) were not much lower than in women in the healthy weight range (26.% as opposed to 31.4%)."

The second proposition, that "IVF is Insufficiently Cost-Effective", Brown highlights that "Claims that the evidence us if sufficient clarity to make decisive cost-effectiveness cutoffs appropriate is disingenuous. Rather, I propose that references to the cost inefficiency of providing IVF to obese people may mask other influences, such as negative attitudes towards obese people that render them easy targets for cost-cutting commissioners."

The final proposition that Brown makes is "the suggestion that those who are responsible for their ill health should be de-prioritised for treatment relative to those who are not responsible for their ill health." Brown highlights that "Given the highly stigmatised nature of obesity, the ambiguity around the status of subfertility as a 'disease', and the confusion around the methodologies used to assess its cost-effectiveness, it is unsurprising that CCGs have chosen to deny IVF treatment to obese people."

Brown then goes on to show that "evidence from diverse research programs including work identifying the social determinants of health and the psychology of behaviour control suggests it is often extremely difficult for individuals to makes changes to the lifestyles that result in significant weight loss. Further, it will often be unclear where a particular individual who is both obese and subfertile is subfertile because of her obesity"

Some smaller studies detailed below also show that BMI has no impact on the outcome of using IVF or ovulation induction.

Vilarino et al.[10] analysed 208 IVF cycles from their clinic and found that there was no correlation between patient BMI and live birth rate.

A study[11] looked at a group of 335 anovulatory women (women who did not ovulate) who were treated with gonadotrophin to induce ovulation. The study found that women with higher BMIs required higher doses of gonadotrophin but that "there was no difference in the rates of ovulation and clinical pregnancy in relation to body weight." Unfortunately, the study only accepted women up to a BMI of 35.

A study[12] in 2010 looked retrospectively at the medical records of 308 women undergoing non-donor IVF and divided into 3 groups based on BMI. There was no significant difference between the three groups in terms of egg quality, implantation or pregnancy rate. They concluded that BMI had no adverse effects on the IVF outcome.

---

[10]Vilarino, F. et al., 2011. Body mass index and fertility: is there a correlation with human reproduction outcomes?. *Gynecological Endocrinology*, [Online]. Volume 27, Issue 4, 232-236. Available at: https://www.tandfonline.com/doi/abs/ 10.3109/09513590.2010.490613?src=recsys&journalCode=igye20 [Accessed 12 February 2019].

[11] Balen, A. et al., 2006. The influence of body weight on response to ovulation induction with gonadotrophins in 335 women with World Health Organization group II anovulatory infertility. *BJOG An Internation Journal of Obstetrics and Gynaecology*, [Online]. Volume113, Issue10 Special Issue: Obesity, 1195-1202. Available at: https:// doi.org/10.1111/j.1471-0528.2006.01034.x [Accessed 3 February 2019].

[12] Sathya, A. et al., 2010. Effect of body mass index on in vitro fertilization outcomes in women. *Journal of Human Reproductive Sciences*, [Online]. Sep-Dec; 3(3), 135-138. Available at: https://www.ncbi.nlm.nih.gov/pmc/articles/PMC3017329/ [Accessed 3 February 2019].

In 2017 Banker et al.[13] conducted a 9-month retrospective study looking at over 2500 women who had undergone IVF and ICSI. They were divided into four groups based on BMI and further subdivided into three groups based on their treatment protocol. Pregnancy rates were found to be unaffected by BMI in all three treatment protocol groups.

You've got this lovely. I know that it can feel scary and a bit weird going in with these questions. After all, it's always been the case that doctors know best. But actually we are the ones who know our bodies best, and we can put ourselves in the position where we can take charge and make the best decisions for us.

---

[13] Banker, M. et al., 2017. Effect of Body Mass Index on the Outcome of In-Vitro Fertilization/Intracytoplasmic Sperm Injection in Women. *Journal of Human Reproductive Sciences*, [Online]. Jan-Mar; 10(1), 37-43. Available at: https://www.ncbi.nlm.nih.gov/pmc/articles/PMC5405646/ [Accessed 3 February 2019].

Chapter 6 - Trusting your body

Just before I started writing this, I caught myself making a batch of pancakes. Not because I was hungry, not for anyone else to eat, just for me to eat because I needed to manage my emotions. Pancakes are my food of choice at the moment (no idea why!?), but I seem to latch onto a particular food that comforts me. For a long time, it was the little scotch pancakes with butter, then it was fairy cakes with coffee icing, I had a small stint on chocolate salted truffles, and now it is the British classic - lemon and sugar pancake.

I find the rhythm of making them therapeutic, going through the same actions and the same routine is calming for me, especially when I'm missing routine in other areas of my life. But then there is the eating. I am not hungry. Not at all. The food I'm going to consume isn't satisfying a physical hunger in me. But it is satisfying a hunger. An emotional hunger, a way of dealing with difficult emotions I have in my life.

Sometimes I can sit with these emotions and process them, but as an introvert, I need space to do that, and with 2 kids, I don't get a lot of space. So right now, my emotional crutch is eating pancakes. What thoughts led me to find comfort in the pancakes? Lots of simple life circumstances building up. I wrote a whole long paragraph about my frustrations (which was very cathartic!), but it boiled down to not getting my needs met. It was really that simple.

So what purpose did the food provide? It filled a hole in me, I don't know where this hole came from or when it started or what is missing? But maybe you feel this hole too? This type of eating is often called emotional eating and has been labelled as bad. But emotional eating is something we learn as babies when we use breastmilk for comfort. We didn't invent it as adults. It's just a different way of coping with the overwhelming world we live in. I know that this food might make my body physically uncomfortable, but I make a choice, is that physical discomfort worth the emotional relief?

Right now, the biggest thing missing from my life is time for me. Time to be me, time to do the things that I want to do and achieve the things I want to achieve. Maybe you are missing that time too? Maybe you feel like you need to fill a hole? Maybe you feel there is a missing piece of your family? Maybe you don't feel understood by anyone around you? All your friends got pregnant really easily and now have kids. You don't feel that you fit in anymore. This hole can completely consume you and take over your life. It can make everything else in your life seem meaningless. As you look at your life you know that there are so many things to be grateful for, but you can't feel it, and you can't see it on a day to day basis because this hole swallows everything up in its wake.

Exercise

Grab a pen and paper or download the "Fat and Fertile" accompanying PDF that contains all the exercises from the book that you can fill in straight on your computer or print off.

Access the PDF at nicolasalmon.co.uk/bookbonus

In the centre of the paper, draw a big circle and a smaller circle inside. This is your hole.

Inside the smallest hole, I want you to write down all the current strategies you use to try and fill this hole that you feel.

For me, it's pancakes (obviously!), sleeping (normally napping when I don't really need to), binging Netflix, scrolling mindlessly on social media to name a few.

Be as specific as you can. If you eat to fill this hole, what specific foods do you eat, and how do you eat them? Is it in secret, standing over the kitchen sink? If it's spending time on your phone, what do you look at?

Inside the bigger circle, I want you to write down how these actions make you feel. What benefit do you get from them?

For me, it's a sensation of fullness from the food, a kind of numbness sometimes, escapism, a lot of these activities kind of take me away from current emotions or moods that I'm feeling.

Really think about what exactly happens when you do these activities and how you feel. I know you might be thinking, well there is actually no benefit from me watching 7 hours of Netflix in a row, but you wouldn't do something unless there was a benefit to you, so dig a little deeper and figure out whatever it is (even if it feels slightly absurd)

In the space around the edge of your circle, I want you to start to brainstorm how you can begin to get the benefits from these actions in other ways.

For example, I sometimes want to numb out because I'm overstimulated. The benefit of numbing out is that it stops me from snapping with all the excess stimulation, so I need to look at other

> ways of avoiding overstimulation - like going to bed earlier and blocking out some solo time regularly.
>
> Maybe you want to numb yourself from the intense grief, sadness or anger you feel at the situation or your body. Giving yourself that numb time is allowing you to continue with life and not to get completely overwhelmed. It's a defence mechanism to allow you to function, maybe not as you'd like but to just get through the day.
>
> So how can you give yourself that respite or relief in another way?

Two really important things to note:

1. Doing all the things I mentioned above aren't bad. I'm not saying you have to stop doing them at all. They are coping strategies, and if they are working, then it is a choice as to whether you use them. The major word being choice! Sometimes it can feel like you do these things on autopilot and that can be really detrimental to your mental health, so let's make it an active choice.

2. Sometimes it is actually ok to feel these emotions and be with them. It can feel scary because we are so used to putting on a mask to get up, go to work and get on with life but you are allowed to be present with these emotions, no matter how unusual that feels.

The T in the FAT+ve Fertility Framework is all about relearning how to trust our bodies and listen to what they need. One of the biggest concerns that women have when they finally begin to release the grip that dieting has had on them their whole life is that they are afraid to eat. Scared that without the diet, they will eat everything and completely lose control. I understand this, but at the same time, it doesn't make any sense. We have been reduced to thinking that we have no control, and we have no power. That we are slaves to our cravings and are addicted to food.

The fear that we have is based on binging episodes we may have experienced in the past. Those episodes were a response to restriction. When we restrict food in our diets, our body panics. It thinks that we are going into a famine. To keep us safe it puts us on red alert. We need to get as much high-calorie, high-fat food as we possibly can. We think about food all the time, and we crave those foods. It's a biological response to our body, thinking that we are in an emergency situation. When we take the restriction away, we take away this response.

Restriction doesn't just come in the form of calorie restriction. Any type of rules you have around eating can impact this. Rules about the types of food you are allowed to eat, when you are allowed to eat, the foods you can and can't eat together, all these rules are external influences telling you what is and isn't ok.

From young children, we are trained to eat when we are told.

"You can't have a snack, it's nearly tea time."
"Finish everything on your plate, and you can have pudding."
"Eat your broccoli and 3 mouthfuls of carrots, or you can't get down from the table."

We are trained out of listening to our bodies about what we want to eat and when we want to eat it. In days gone by, there were very practical reasons for this. Food was scarcer, so choice and availability was limited. But that's not the case anymore. Yet we are left with a culture that gives no credibility to our natural hunger, natural satiety and choice around food in any given moment.

My boys are three and five. I'm being extremely mindful about how I talk about food with them, but this shit is so ingrained in me, I have to catch myself so many times. Obviously, I want them to eat food that will support them to grow and feel healthy. I want that for myself too, but I'm not willing to force them to stop listening to their bodies about when they are hungry, when they are full and what they want to eat. This is a delicate balance, if I left it up to Sebby, he would eat ice cream all day, and I would feel like I'd completely failed as a parent. But what would happen if I let them eat what they wanted?

I remember reading a slightly sarcastic article ages ago about the parents who said yes. It was very biased and painted these parents as hippy types who were too lazy to parent and let their kids run rings around them. The basic premise of the article is that they let them eat whatever they wanted, and sure when the experiment first started, they ate ice cream until they were sick. But once they realised they had control, they could choose and weren't limited by their parents, they begin to eat a varied diet, without being forced to eat their vegetables and without being sent to bed without dinner. They listened to their body and chose the food they needed in each given moment.

How much of our food choices are about control? When you are trying to get pregnant, you want to control the process. So many women I speak to would be happy (ish!) to wait if they just knew that in 3 years they would have their family. If they could only control the outcome. That's why this whole baby making process completely takes over your life. You have absolutely no control over when you get pregnant. So you feel like you need to take control of other things. Things that you feel like you can control to a certain extent. Like your food choices, like your lifestyle decisions, how much coffee you drink, how many runs you do, what supplements you take. Having this control gives you the sense that you are doing everything you can to make this happen. The guilt lessens slightly because it's not your fault, right? You are doing it all.

How much of what you decide to eat comes from a place of restriction and control? Control is when my secret eating habit started. When I was fifteen, I was on some diet (who know which one now!) It was pretty restrictive, and you could have either a red day or a green day (something to do with mixing carbs and proteins I think but who the fuck cares anymore). My food was controlled at home, and I brought my lunch to school. But on the walk from the bus to school each and every day I walked past a sweet shop, and every day I would go in there, buy chocolate toffee and scoff the lot on the ten-minute walk to school. No one ever saw me do this. It was my secret.

It gave me control back over my diet. That control about what to eat had been completely taken away. I was a good girl. I didn't want to upset my parents, but I so desperately wanted to control something in my life, and that something became the sugar that I wasn't allowed to eat at home. Have you ever eaten in secret? Why did you feel like you needed to hide it? What restrictions do you place on your eating now? How do these restrictions make you feel? What benefit are they giving you?

I want to tell you about my current situation with food. I kind of imagine myself in a middle place right now, a sort of food limbo. I don't weight myself, and I don't diet. I allow myself to eat whatever I want, whenever I want. I'm not perfect. I still worry about food sometimes and find myself being triggered by having certain foods in the house.

For the longest time, I didn't allow myself to have "bad" foods in the house as a strategy for not eating them. Recently my husband came home with a couple of tubs of ice cream, and I was livid with him. The reason? The belief I held about myself was that I would eat any sugary foods in the house until nothing was left. That I would eat and eat them until I was sick. That's not what happened though - they are still in the freezer - but it triggered off that fear in me that I would go on a massive binge and I couldn't trust myself.

I still need to watch my language around food. I avoid labelling food as good or bad or anything except factually what it is. And I am really gentle with myself with my choices around food. I try to listen to what I need and pay attention to when I'm hungry and when I'm full. That's it and for me right now - it's enough.

I'm not perfect, but I want to outline some steps for you to try to move slowly away from the fear of food and the belief that you cannot trust yourself around food. I want you to find peace and joy in food once again. Food can be joyful. So much of our social lives and celebration is around food. You don't have to miss out on going to a wedding, or enjoying a piece of birthday cake, or missing dinner with your friends because there is nothing you can eat. I spent many social events worried about what I wanted to eat, what I should eat and what I had eaten, rather than enjoying the company of the people I was with. If you need some extra support with your relationship with food, you can sign up for my 8-week support program called The Fertility UnDiet.

Exercise

Grab a pen and paper or download the "Fat and Fertile" accompanying PDF that contains all the exercises from the book that you can fill in straight on your computer or print off.

Access the PDF at nicolasalmon.co.uk/bookbonus

Throughout the day, before each time you eat something, I want you to ask yourself 3 questions.

Will this food help me thrive or survive?

2. What impact will this food have on my physical and mental body?

3. What benefit will this food give me?

The purpose of these questions is not to stop you from eating the food or to find a reason for you to beat yourself up for eating the food.

It's to bring awareness and curiosity to the act of eating. As children, we knew when our bodies were hungry and what we wanted to eat, but we've been trained to discard that internal voice and instead eat based on arbitrary meal times and foods that "should" be eaten at a particular time.

Will this food help me thrive or survive?

This isn't another way of labelling good or bad food. I want you to look at the food at that particular moment and decide if the food is going to add anything to your life? Is it going to help you thrive in some way? The same food might help you thrive one day and not another. The same food might help your friend thrive but has no real impact for you. This isn't a judgement of the food itself but what impact you think it's going to have on you right now.

2. What impact will this food have on my physical and mental body?

Taking question 1 a little deeper. How is this food going to affect me? Will it impact my digestion? Will it affect my sleep later? Will it improve my energy? Will it alter my mood? Understanding the impact that food has on your body is where the big bucks are. Listening to feedback from your body is where you will begin to unravel what foods are best for you.

(Journalling is my fav way to do this - check out my Nurture Fertility Journal) When you fully understand the impact a food will have on you, you can truly make an informed decision about whether you want to eat it.

3. What benefit will this food give me?

Taking question 2 deeper still, look at which of the impacts are of benefit to you? Maybe you get more energy. Maybe the sensation of eating it gives you pleasure. Maybe the act of sharing it with your friend brings you joy. Maybe the foods make you feel satiated. Notice what benefits you are going to get from the food.

This awareness allows you to decide, really decide if you want to eat the food. It may take a little while to get into this habit (and if you forget, just start where you are) but soon it will be an automatic response rather than an intentional thought process. Soon every mouthful you take will be decided upon how good this food will make you feel. You'll naturally stop eating when you are done, and you will find peace with food. Food is there for your benefit. It's there to provide the building blocks for your body to grow and to repair. It's there to give you the energy to move your body and grow your baby.

So let's take it one step at a time. Grab your journal and begin to get curious about the effect that every food has on your body.

How to Journal

If you haven't done much journaling in your life, now is a great time to start. It's a reflective practice so the more you do, the more you get out of it. If you love pretty stationary, definitely check out my Nurture Fertility Journal. But you don't need anything fancy to start, just a pen and paper. There are lots of ways to journal, you can reflect on the day in the evening or the following morning, or do it as you go. The best way is the easiest way for you.

Track the things that are most important to you. Here are some ideas.

Sleep - quantity and quality.
Food - what you are eating and when.
Mood - how you're feeling through the day
Energy - how your energy varies throughout the day
Signs and symptoms - how you feel in your body
Hydration - how much water you're drinking
Movement - when and how you move your body

Other exercises you can include:

Gratitude - write down three specific things you're grateful for that day
A phrase or affirmation that resonates with you
5 minutes of free writing. This is writing about whatever is on your mind, or you can use prompts such as 'what went well today?', 'what do I need to let go of' or 'how can I be kind to myself?'

Repairing your relationship with food

It was only once I was out of the dieting yo-yo-ing phase of my life, that I understood my eating disorder. I had no idea I even had an eating disorder up until this point. Dieting was just the normal thing that everyone did, right? When you hear eating disorder - you think anorexia or bulimia, thin women who have body dysmorphia. But eating disorders extend far further than that. Anyone can suffer from an eating disorder, average-sized women, men, even fat women.

Eating disorders often start with disordered eating. A place where you are restricting your food and eating, not based on hunger, but from a place of fear.

Fear of what the food will do to your body. Fear of what people will think of what you're eating or what you look like. Here are some signs that you have a disordered view of food and your body.

- Your self worth is dependent on the food you consume and what your body looks like.
- You get really anxious when you have to eat in public or at social events.
- You obsessively count calories or portions or macronutrients or anything else that defines a particular food as good or bad.
- You have strict routines or rituals around foods.

An eating disorder takes that further still with all these behaviours becoming more extreme.

The trigger for me was showing someone else what I was eating. It was innocent enough. I asked my sister-in-law (who is a nurse in an exercise rehabilitation centre) what kind of eating plans they use. She said she'd be happy to show me how it works and just to write down what I'm eating for a week, then we could go over it. That's when the fear set in. Logically I knew that she wouldn't shame me for my food or make me feel guilty for what I was eating, but I was still ashamed of writing it all down and showing it to her. Ashamed it meant that I wasn't good enough. Afraid that I should be doing better. Scared of what she would think of me. It made no logical sense, and that's when I knew that years of disordered eating had given me an eating disorder. It was only once I was able to understand that such a thing could even exist for a woman of my size that I could grasp the damage years of dieting had done to my relationship with food.

Choose food from a place of love and the intention to nourish your body. Intention is everything. With every mouthful, with every supplement, set the intention that this food is making your body strong and healthy.

Repairing your relationship with exercise

Exercise can play a huge role in the way that we nourish our bodies, but so often in the past, we have used it as a form of punishment. This was my story until a couple of years ago. At the beginning of 2018, my cycles were lengthening again. I had two 100+ day menstrual cycles in a row, and I was miserable. We weren't trying to conceive, but I was desperate to get more in tune with my body's natural rhythms and I was getting more and more frustrated with my body.

Then I started exercising regularly three times a week because I loved it. Within the first three months, my menstrual cycles reduced to 35, 47 and 31 days. It speaks for itself, exercise is powerful. But I'll be completely honest, this is the first time in my life I have ever enjoyed exercise. I just thought I wasn't one of those people. You know the one, always in activewear talking about their latest 10k or marathon or Ironman. I could not understand the appeal, why would anyone spend so much time exercising?

Because for me, exercise equalled punishment. There was absolutely no other reason I could see to move your body than if you'd eaten too much cake and needed to lose weight. But yet again, I really had no idea that exercise wasn't going to help me lose weight. It's great for loads of things but purely weight loss? Not so much. In my head, if I forced myself to exercise regularly, it gave me a free pass to eat what I wanted. So interspersed between the diets were bouts at the gym, boot camp and any other intense exercise I could try to help me lose the weight.

I hated exercising in public, my breasts felt too big, and I felt so self-conscious in any kind of sportswear, I was convinced everyone was laughing at me behind my back, and I felt like that was my punishment. Almost like being in the stocks in the Middle Ages. Paraded around for all to see - this is what happens when you inhale Dairy Milk chocolate. So I endured it, but it only deepened my hatred for my body. How could I ever learn to love this blob of fat that everyone laughs at?

I don't think it helped that exercise was always forced upon me. I wasn't sporty at school, PE was always something I endured rather than enjoyed. I still have memories of dredging around the cross country course on a rainy and muddy day, secretly discussing how we could get away with shortcuts. My first real body shame experience was from my secondary school PE teacher. I went to a pretty strict school, and our PE uniform was short gym skirts, PE knickers (whose invention was PE knickers?) and a school polo shirt. Lots of the other athletic girls wore black cycling shorts under their skirts (makes sense right!) the first time I did this, my teacher told me to take them off because my legs were too fat and it made me look too masculine.

So how did I go from doing no exercise consistently ever, to working out 3 times a week and loving it? Once it clicked, it was simple. I just had to change my intention. I didn't move my body to lose weight, I started because I want to be able to keep up with my very active boys. I want to be the mum who goes on all the adventures and isn't afraid to try things, I don't want to be left on the sidelines, too afraid that my bum is going to get stuck in the rollercoaster seat (#truestory)

My intention was one of nourishing not punishing my body, and that's when the game changed. I'm excited to learn how to lift weights, do handstands and move my body. I feel like athletic achievements are no longer just not meant for me. I discovered that I can move my body however I damn well please and finding what feels good to me (and not what burns the most calories) is essential.

I also learnt to be kind. Not only in how I move my body, but when and how often. Women are cyclical, our bodies naturally change throughout our menstrual cycle, and so does our nutritional requirements and our movement. Moving your body in the same way during ovulation and your period will feel (and should feel) completely different. You are not a lazy and will-less pig if you don't feel like exercising at particular times of the month, it's completely normal. You haven't failed if you miss a day at the gym because you don't feel like moving your body, it's ok.

For a quick rule of thumb-

Menstruation (D1-5 roughly - when you are bleeding) is great for resting. If you want to move, try slow, gentle exercise like yoga.

Follicular phase (roughly D6-13 of a 28-day cycle - before ovulation) is fantastic for cardio this is when you'll generally have the most energy.

Ovulation (D14-16) is when you'll feel great but don't do too much (you'll be tempted as you'll feel like superwoman) and you may even need a rest day or 2 when ovulating.

Luteal phase (D17-end) is great for strength training.

This is a rough idea of what works well in the different phases, NOT what works well for you. Track your exercise and how you feel about it against your cycle day and see what patterns you notice. Maybe you always need a rest day on D25? If you have irregular cycles, maybe you notice that you love going to spin 3 days in a row before ovulation.

Working out what movement feels good for you and when is a great way to get in touch with your body and begin to enjoy exercise. Find what feels good.

It always comes back to this. Find a way to move your body that feels joyful, that feels playful, that is exciting and feels good. It really is that simple and not be afraid to keep trying until you find it.

It could be ballet (yes fat people can do ballet) swimming, kickboxing, line dancing, weight lifting, yoga, BMX-ing, Pilates, running, walking, climbing, hoop dancing, cycling, diving .... whatever it is, love it!

Chapter 7 - Your beliefs around being fat

What do you believe about fat women? The media likes to tell fat women what we are meant to think about ourselves. We are meant to believe that our bodies are shameful. We are meant to believe that we always need to be on the lookout for the next fad diet that is going to fix us. We are meant to believe that we should be punishing ourselves with gruelling exercise regimens. We are meant to believe that we are second class citizens, treated differently from those who have socially acceptable bodies.

What do you believe about yourself as a fat woman? Maybe all the above apply, and maybe none of them do. It doesn't matter. What matters is what you believe. Do you believe that your weight or your health is impacting your ability to get pregnant? Do you believe that you should be treated differently based on your size? Do you believe that you deserve less or are worth less than others who are thinner than you?

Creating a positive mindset is a big part of the FAT+ve fertility framework. It's more than just forcing yourself to think happy thoughts all the time. Your beliefs and the thoughts going around your head every day play a huge role in your mental health and your physical health. We are going to examine what your beliefs are and how we can alter them to help us feel better in our bodies and get pregnant faster.

Exercise

I'd like you to take a minute and really think about what being a fat woman means to you.

Grab a pen and paper or download the "Fat and Fertile" accompanying PDF that contains all the exercises from the book that you can fill in straight on your computer or print off. Access the PDF at nicolasalmon.co.uk/bookbonus

Write down and complete the statement "I believe that, as a fat woman....... "

Keep going until you have at least 20 lines completed. It will be hard to get to 20. You'll say, "I'm done" but keep writing, because every belief that comes out, whether you know it or not, is affecting how you live your life on a day-to-day basis.

These conscious AND unconscious beliefs are making your decisions. They are choosing what you eat, how you show up in the world and most importantly, how you feel.

Here is what came up for me when I first did this exercise, in case you get stuck and need a prompt.

I believe that, as a fat woman, I can't get pregnant.
I believe that, as a fat woman, I can't wear a swimsuit.
I believe that, as a fat woman, I can't wear the latest fashions.
I believe that, as a fat woman, I can't go to the spa.
I believe that, as a fat woman, I can't eat food in public.
I believe that, as a fat woman, I can't travel on public transport.

Your beliefs around being fat

I believe that, as a fat woman, I can't go to a yoga class.
I believe that, as a fat woman, I can't be a good mother.
I believe that, as a fat woman, I can't shop on the high street.
I believe that, as a fat woman, I can't wear beautiful clothes.
I believe that, as a fat woman, no-one will love me.
I believe that, as a fat woman, I'm not pretty.
I believe that, as a fat woman, I'm disgusting.
I believe that, as a fat woman, I'm really unhealthy.
I believe that, as a fat woman, I'm going to get diabetes.
I believe that, as a fat woman, I'm going to die young.
I believe that, as a fat woman, I'm not worthy of nice things.
I believe that, as a fat woman, I can't be successful in my career.
I believe that, as a fat woman, I don't deserve a family.

So where the hell did these beliefs come from and how can we shift them?

The first step to shifting these beliefs is recognising that they are there, so well done for uncovering them and digging deep to get a long list. If you skipped the exercise thinking you'll do it later, DO IT NOW. Get your phone and write it down. It will take you 10 minutes max, and if you don't do it now, you will not do it.

The next step is figuring out where we got these beliefs. More often than not, we inherit these beliefs from others. We don't just wake up one day and think that all fat girls are lazy pigs. Beliefs can come from anywhere. It may be something you picked up in childhood, it may be a passing comment a friend said or a quip your doctor made at your expense.

For each belief on your list, write down any thoughts that spring to mind about where it came from. Does it bring up any memories for you? Do you remember anyone saying that to you? How does this belief make you feel? When was the first time you felt like that?

Your beliefs are not you

I want to share something with you that completely changed my life. It was the catalyst that helped me see the world for more than just what lay on the surface. For more than just what shows we watch on TV, gossiping with my colleagues or worrying about what I looked like. This one thing helped me see that my life could be so much more than these superficial things.

Your beliefs are not you. You can change your beliefs.

It took me a while to actually understand this, but once I realised that I could change my beliefs and my thoughts then the whole world opened up before my eyes. I used to think that everyone had the same beliefs (or at least everyone I knew) and that everyone thought the same things. Everyone lived the same life plus or minus a few minor details, like what music you liked or your favourite movies. But it's not true.

We now live in a world where you can see and experience so much more of what life has to offer, and even that is only the tip of the iceberg. We live in a generation where so much information is at our fingertips, you can find out the mating rituals of the white-spotted pufferfish, that the tongue is the strongest muscle in the body and that more lifeforms are living on your skin than people on the planet. With the touch of a button, you can read any book that has ever been published and expand your mind in a million different ways.

You can change how you see the world and how you think about it. But most people don't. Most people use the internet to cement their current beliefs further (that and watch cute cat videos on youtube!)

Every single second you're alive, you are taking in thousands upon thousands of bits of information Even as you are sitting here reading this book, your eyes are taking in every single aspect of your surroundings, your ears are picking up every sound, your nose, every smell, your fingers, the different sensations of the surface you're touching. 11 million various bits of information per second. The problem with this is that your brain cannot process all those bit of information, it's impossible to handle, and for the most part, it's a waste of resources.

So we filter. We filter big style. Our conscious mind processes on average, 50 of the 11 million possible bits of data. And how does it know which parts to filter? It uses your beliefs. So if you believe that as a fat woman, you can't get pregnant, your brain will filter the magazine you're reading to support that and filter out information that doesn't support that belief. Your beliefs are strengthened by the evidence that you find. But it's biased because the contrary evidence isn't even flagged up in your consciousness? So if everything you are filtering is running through your beliefs, how on earth can you change them?

The very first step is awareness. Being aware of your beliefs and these filters means that you will begin to notice when you are using them. You can stop yourself and think, actually is this true? You can also bring awareness to your thoughts around it. Challenge yourself to really think about the opposite aspect to an idea or opinion that you have. This expands your awareness and really helps you see beyond your normal vision.

Try something new. Read books that you've never thought of reading before, watch films from a different culture, listen to different music. Allow yourself to experience the world in someone else's shoes. By letting yourself see different perspectives on topics that interest you, you can begin to understand that you have a choice about what you think. Only by seeing the millions of different options are you in a position to decide what you actually want to think and believe.

If you only ever tasted vanilla ice-cream, it would be your favourite. It's only fair that you get to taste every flavour of ice cream before you pick your real favourite. And sometimes you may want to change your mind, maybe you fancy mint choc chip instead of caramel fudge brownie today but if you didn't know that mint choc chip existed then you'd never try it.

Giving yourself permission to change your mind is important too. It's how we grow and learn. We are never going to know it all, and that's OK. As women, we feel the need to be perfect and to do everything perfectly, but you know what, we can only do our best with what we know right now. We will learn more and things will change, but we can't beat ourselves up for not knowing things sooner or not doing things differently because we did the best we knew how to.

If we had waited or didn't do anything, then nothing would get done, and we'd be in a state of constant stress and anxiety waiting for the perfect time. There is never a perfect time, do it now!

So the question now is not, "what do you believe?" because that's in the past. The question now is, what do you want to believe? Isn't that an exciting question! You can believe anything you want about yourself, literally anything. So what are you going to choose? What do you want to believe about yourself

so erm yep as soon as the infinite possibilities come up your mind goes blank.

......nothing........

Literally every other minute of the day, your mind is racing with crappy thoughts, you cannot turn off the outpouring of crazy things you think about. It's OK love, it's completely normal. So let's start really small. What do you need right now? Right in this moment. What do you need? What will help you feel better about yourself, help you move through the day, help you sleep tonight?

Your beliefs around being fat

Once you've thought of that one thing that you need right now, go ahead and do it. I'll wait here. OK? Done? Great. Now how did that make you feel? Do you want to continue to feel like that? If so, awesome, if not, why not?

You know what I know about you right now? You are someone who takes care of themselves. You see what you did there ↑, you figured about what you needed and you took care of business. That is someone who takes care of themselves.

(And if you didn't do the thing.....GO DO THE THING!)

Do you believe that about yourself? Beliefs are tricky, sometimes you can flip them in an instant, and sometimes they take a while to really cement in. After all, you are rewiring your brain.

It's like a park. Your regular thoughts and beliefs walk the same way every day and they slowly over time have created paths (or deep trenches in some cases!) which it's easy for you to fall into. It takes a little bit more work to walk on the grass and find a new way to go, and it might take a few days/weeks/months before this path feels familiar like the old one did.

So this new belief - you are someone who takes care of themselves. What do you think that looks like on a day-to-day basis? Is there someone in your life (someone you know or someone you admire) who is really good at taking care of themselves? Like they really own it, unapologetically just put their needs first and take excellent care of themselves. What does that look like? What habits do they do every day? How do they talk about themselves? What boundaries do they have in place?

Now you are you, and I don't want you to think that you have to "do" anyone else, but it can be fascinating to see what it is about this person that personifies that belief for you. Write down everything you can think of that comes to mind about how this person takes care of themselves.

Now you get to decide what is going to work for you.

What habits would you like to do every day to take care of you?
How do you want to talk about yourself in a caring way?
How are you going to think about yourself in a caring way?
What boundaries do you want to put in place to make sure that your needs come first?

This may look like a lot, and you might be thinking, "Woah there Nelly", that's a lot to change! But don't worry about that right now, think about in dreamland, how you would integrate this belief into your life so that people look at you and think "wow she takes excellent care of herself."

The next question I want you to think about is, how can this be easy? How can you make these habits so easy that's it's actually more difficult not to do them than it is to do them? Pick one or two to start with. We'll start with an easy one.

Say you wanted to drink more water. Staying hydrated is a really great way to take care of yourself. You wake up and have a glass already on the table (you put it there the night before), so you see it straight away, fill it and start the day with a big glass of water. You have a refillable bottle by the sink, and while you're there, you fill it up and put it in your bag, so you've got some water for your commute to walk. As you walk into the office, you refill your bottle and put it on your desk. It's always in your sight, so you drink regularly. Because you are so well hydrated, you need a wee and every time you go to the loo, you refill your water bottle so that you always have water when you need it.

Your beliefs around being fat

You see how this becomes second nature when you make it easy for yourself? By doing just a couple of things the night before you are setting yourself up for success and you can apply this method to anything.

Want to go for a run in the morning? Put all your workout clothes by your bed the night before.

Want to eat more nutritious food? Plan your meals and spend a couple of hours doing meal prep at the weekend.

We want to start small with any new habits you decide to implement. Don't try to change everything at once. Why? Your brain isn't designed that way.

Your brain has three main parts, the oldest part of your brain at the back, the middle part and the biggest part at the front. The oldest part of your brain - the reptilian brain - is responsible for keeping you alive. It's in charge of making sure that you keep breathing and stay out of danger. This part of your brain does not think logically, well actually it almost thinks too logically.

It goes like this: You have stayed alive so far, doing precisely what you've been doing right? Making any significant changes is unpredictable, therefore higher risk of death; therefore, we definitely don't want to do that. This is the reason why big life changes are so hard to stick to. Your brain is working against you, and it will do anything to stay alive. So how can we trick this part of our brain into letting make the changes that we want to in our lives? It's about micro-habits. Tiny, tiny steps that you can take every day to get you to where you want to be.

My definition of a micro-habit has 2 components:

It's not scary. It does not fill you with dread at the thought of doing it. So if for example, you wanted to run a marathon, you wouldn't start with a habit of running an hour every day, you would start with walk/running for 10 minutes (or whatever is not scary for you!). When you get out there, you may want to go a bit longer, but the point isn't to trick yourself into running further. It's to get your out of the door and build up that non-scary goal.

It takes less than 15 minutes. Making sure that your habits are short means that you are much less likely to avoid doing them. Even if it's the end of the day and you remember just before bed, you can handle 15 minutes, right? As above you can always do more, but that isn't the point.

We want these habits to stick. We want to make them easy and part of who we are. So that we are the person who takes care of herself. Using micro-habits is the perfect way to motivate yourself to keep these habits up. Use a habit tracker to mark down each habit you complete every day. Not breaking the chain of crosses is actually an excellent motivator. And you have the evidence right before your eyes that you are taking care of yourself each and every day.

Download the "Fat and Fertile" accompanying PDF that contains all the exercises from the book and a handy habit tracker that you can fill in straight on your computer or print off. Access the PDF at nicolasalmon.co.uk/bookbonus

NOTE: A habit tracker is not another stick to beat yourself up with. You know what women who look after themselves also do? Give themselves a fucking break! They realise that life happens, and while we want to maintain these habits for our health, we do not want to do that at the expense of our mental health. So track away but remember gaps are just as important for our health as a complete tracker.

What else do you want to believe about yourself? "I take care of myself" is one which I think most of us will want to believe (but these are your beliefs so feel free to change it/dump it if it doesn't feel right for you.) but now you get to go crazy. Think about the kind of person you want to be (you are probably already most of the way there and don't even know it yet), how you want to feel on a daily basis, the people you want to spend time with, the difference you want to make in this world.

Exercise

Grab a pen and paper or download the "Fat and Fertile" accompanying PDF that contains all the exercises from the book that you can fill in straight on your computer or print off. Access the PDF at nicolasalmon.co.uk/bookbonus

Write "I want to believe" in the middle, set a timer for 15 minutes and go nuts. See what comes up for you.

It's only a small step from "I want to believe" to "I believe."

Five steps to changing those beliefs

1. Decide what you want to believe about yourself.
2. Think about someone in your life who already has that belief. How do they show up?
3. Decide what daily habits you want to create to support that belief.
4. Make them easy for yourself. Pick one or two and start small.

5. Change your thoughts. When you catch yourself thinking the old belief (and you will, it's so normal to follow those old paths), notice the thought, mentally say "stop that's not helpful" and flip it to your new belief.

Thoughts are a big part of your beliefs. Your beliefs are like the blueprint of a house, the reference guide to the bigger picture. Your thoughts are the materials, the bricks, the cement, the ...(running out of building metaphors here) and your actions are the building of the house. If you've got the blueprint right, you'll buy the right materials, but if blueprint doesn't match what you want your house to look like, then you'll end up with the wrong house.

All your thoughts stem from what you believe about the world, and most of them fall into three categories.

The past - thinking about something that has already happened, replaying things in your mind, what you should have done, what went wrong, thinking about what an awful person you are etc.
The present - worrying about things going on right now
The future - worrying about things that haven't happened yet.

In our heads, we spend a lot of time in the past and the future and surprisingly little time in the present. We are either worrying about what has already happened or stressing about what's coming up. Both of these pastimes are pretty fruitless, we cannot change the past, and we cannot predict the future. Being able to be more present in your life is a really helpful way of making life more enjoyable.

A classic example is food. For so much of my life, 90% of my thoughts were about food. I worried about what I had already eaten and what that meant about me as a person. I panicked about what was to come and what I should eat for the rest of the day to get back on track. If I'd fucked it up for that day, I thought about what I could binge eat until I got back on the wagon tomorrow. I worried about what the scales would say the next time I stood on them. I worried about what other people were thinking of me if I was eating or not eating. Basically, it was all about food. Worrying about what I'd already eaten and worrying about what I was going to eat. I was so enveloped in this world, there wasn't much room for anything else.

I didn't think about how good the food tasted after the first mouthful. I didn't notice when I was hungry or when I was full. All the actual pleasure from the food was not there. All the signals my body was sending me, were completely ignored. I was living in my head and completely disconnected from my body.

It was a slow journey from the place of being consumed by food to where I am now. And where I am right now is not perfect, but I've learnt that it doesn't have to be. I don't get a gold star for eating all the "right" food. No-one is going to come along and give me the prize for the world's healthiest eater. The only person I'm doing this for is me. So what happened, how did I get from there to here?

I made a decision. I looked at the evidence. I looked at the piles of diet books on my bookcase. The army of habits I'd created from the advice of some expert or other. I looked at my body. Diets didn't work. So that's when I made myself two promises. I was never going to weigh myself again. I was never going to diet again. I changed my beliefs and thoughts.

Once I'd made those decisions, it freed up so much mental space for me. I was no longer worried about the number on the scales because I was never going to see it again. It was never going to stare back at me in that judging straight lined electric number way that only scales can. I was no longer wasting my time researching the next diet that was sure to work (not!). I didn't have to plan my calories or portion sizes meticulously.

So instead of believing that I had to change my size before I could do things. I just started doing the things. I no longer believed that my weight was holding me back. Sure there were a million different hiccups. Daily thoughts were trying to tempt me over to the dark side.

"But look, Nicola, look how fat you look in this photo. You definitely need to get back to dieting."

"But what about intermittent fasting? That's not a diet. You could do that to lose weight."

"Your clothes don't even fit. You are such a fat pig."

And on it went. But I kept my promises to myself, and when I spotted these unhelpful thoughts, I said no thank you and got on with my day. I changed my behaviours. Once the beliefs were laid, it became so much easier to look after my body in the way that I wanted to. For the first time, I believed that my body was worth taking care of, so it became my priority.

That's right. The first thing on my list. Not after work, family, friends, the very first thing. Do you know what happened? I started enjoying moving my body. I found a new love of weight-lifting. I started leaving things on my plate when I was full. I skipped a meal if I wasn't hungry. I ate double portions if I was starving. And I didn't judge myself on any of my behaviours. I just accepted that at that moment, I was nourishing my body and wellbeing in the way that it needed. If I can do it, so can you.

But how does all this help you get pregnant?

Changing your beliefs around your body and getting pregnant is going to have a huge impact on how you show up for your body every day. So many fertility experts talk about fertility as if being fertile is a higher level of health. But that's not the truth. Your reproductive system is just another reflection of your general health. Your reproductive system isn't separate from your body like you see in the biology textbooks. Your ovaries, uterus, vagina are all mushed in there with the rest of your organs and they all impact on each other.

Making positive steps in a (seemingly unrelated) area of your health will impact all of your health. Your sleep will affect your mood. Your movement habits will affect your energy. How often you poo will affect your hormones. It's all interlinked. Our bodies are more intelligent than we can even begin to comprehend. If we give them the right tools, by listening to what they tell us, then all the different components will work in perfect harmony. All it takes is us to listen to them and follow our guts - literally!

Your menstrual cycle

Relearning and trusting your body goes way beyond the food you eat and how you move. Every month (or longer or shorter depending on where you're at right now) your hormones change and flow in a predictable pattern. It might not always feel predictable, and if you have irregular cycles, it might be very far from predictable right now. But your body is designed to have a monthly cycle.

Hormones are a funny old thing. We are taught the basics at high school but never really told what impact they actually have on our lives. I remember drawing a graph in high school biology showing how the hormones went up and down over a month, but I had absolutely no idea what that meant for me, especially as I wasn't even having regular periods (thanks PCOS!).

The truth is that our hormones have a HUGE impact on our daily lives (duh!) They affect what foods our body wants, our appetite, the way we want to move our body, our energy, our mood and pretty much every other part of your life. When I knew this - so much of my life made sense. It explained why some days at work, I was completely unmotivated to do anything, whereas some days I felt like superwoman and did five days worth of work in one. It explained why I wanted to eat everything in sight in the days leading up to my period. And it finally explained why it was so bloody difficult for me to stick with a significant lifestyle change. How on earth can you be expected to stick to a regular food or exercise regime when your body's requirements change on a daily basis?

Knowing that I wasn't crazy was a big relief. Realising that the seemingly random bouts of low energy and low mood weren't random at all changed my life around. Women aren't erratic beings like we are led to believe. We are actually very regular and reliable - just in our own way, a cyclical way. Once you start to track things based on where you are in your cycle, things start to make sense and patterns begin to show. This information is priceless as it's your own personal health manual. Having this information not only allows you to see what's going on every month but it lets you predict things for the next month.

You'll have the heads up for the days when you're going to feel exhausted (don't plan big social events then!). You'll know when you're a going to feel on fire so you can plan interviews and important dates then. This is the very core of self-care.

If you don't have a regular cycle, you might be thinking, what about me? I'm here with you and it can be frustrating as hell not knowing what your cycle is doing but tracking your cycle is just as (maybe even more) important for you. With irregular cycles, it's often the first part of the cycle (the follicular phase - from the start of your period until ovulation) that varies in length and the second part (the luteal phase - from ovulation until the beginning of your next period) is pretty regular.

Learning how to know when you're ovulating not only helps you in the baby making stakes but also gives you a heads up for roughly when your period will be. And all the other info you uncover will help you figure out what is going on with your hormones and how to help regulate your cycle.

Chapter 8 - Respecting your body

"Why are you fat?"

If anyone has ever asked you why you are fat before, I bet your answer looked something like this:

- I just love chocolate, I can't stop eating sugar.
- I don't know why I put weight on easily, and it's tough for me to lose.
- I'm rubbish at exercising.

We all have our reasons. The things we say to people to excuse the socially unacceptable fact that you are fat. Fat is such a loaded word. When someone asks you this question, you know that's a thinly veiled insult, and you must give an acceptable answer for why on earth your body is in this state, quickly followed by what exactly you are doing to remedy the situation.

For example, "I really struggle to lose weight, but I've just joined this great new liquid-only diet, and they guarantee you lose 7kg in 2 weeks!"

It's not acceptable for you to be happy exactly as you are. That really fucks with people's minds, and they are sure that you are lying to them, that you couldn't possibly find happiness and health in the body that you're currently in.

I want to turn this question on its head. What if being fat is useful for you right now?

"Whaaaaaaaaaaaaat!" I know, I know, that's exactly what you are yelling at me right now.

Everything we do, we do it for a reason. Whether we know what that reason is or not (the subconscious is a powerful thing!), every thought and every action we take has a purpose.

Maybe your fat is protecting you.

In this patriarchal society, women's bodies have been objectified to the extreme. We, as women, have the right to be seen as human and not just some piece of meat to look at. By layering up the fat, you are essentially protecting yourself from being objectified in the same way.

Is there a reason why you want to protect yourself? Did something happen in the past that caused you to want to hide away? This may be an issue to need to explore more in coaching or counselling, but it's important to recognise if your fat is protecting you from the outside world in some way.

Maybe food is your coping mechanism.

When the world gets too tough, we all need a coping mechanism. It is totally normal that food is a comforting habit. When we were babies, we suckled our mother's breast for comfort. It is an entirely natural response. In other cultures, it is completely normal for children up to 3/4 to continue breastfeeding in this way. Maybe by creating a society where extended breastfeeding is abnormal, we are setting up our children to comfort themselves using food in other ways.

If food is your coping mechanism and it calms you down, imagine taking that away cold turkey. Imagine being in a world where you have no coping mechanism. Without a coping mechanism, life feels much harder.

Maybe it's how you nourish and look after yourself.

When I was growing up, sweet food was a treat for me. That meant that chocolate and sweet things were something you got when you were especially good, a way to acknowledge that you were a good girl. It makes complete sense that you might use food to treat yourself and make yourself feel good. This could be you just looking after yourself and loving yourself.

Others do the same thing. I gave up sugar once for six weeks, and it was incredible the responses I had when I refused food that others wanted to give me. Some people were visibly offended that I didn't want to eat a piece of cake that they'd made. The fact that I didn't eat it actually hurt their feelings. It's crazy that my diet had such a significant impact on their mood. Food is a big part of how we look after others as well as ourselves.

Maybe your body is healing.

After years of restrictive eating, your body may need more calories to recover from the restriction. This is a perfectly normal response. When you start to give your body and your brain the freedom to eat what it needs, it may surprise you. You may eat all the chocolate for what feels like forever but give your body the opportunity to reset. It's like a swinging pendulum, it may need to go back the other way to compensate before it comes to rest.

So what does food mean to you? How is being fat benefiting you now? How can you appreciate all the ways your body has been doing the best it can for you?

Nicola Salmon

You are perfect exactly as you are

For the longest time, I believed that my fat meant that I was less than. Less than in so many ways.

My fat meant I wasn't pretty. No-one found fat girls pretty. Pretty girls were worth more than me. My fat meant I wasn't smart. If I couldn't do something as simple as losing weight, that must mean I'm dumb. Smart girls were worth more than me. My fat meant I wasn't lovable. My family were constantly trying to change me. I know now that they were doing it precisely because they loved me but back when I was younger, them wanting to change me meant I wasn't good enough exactly how I was. Because I wasn't skinny like my sister, we were treated differently, and it seemed to me that my love depended on if I lost weight or what size my clothes were.

Do you feel less than?

Maybe right now to you, your fat means that you are not worthy of getting pregnant. You are not worthy of becoming a mother You are not healthy enough to get pregnant. You are too fat to get pregnant. Your doctor won't give you tests to see what's going on with your fertility. You aren't eligible for IVF.

These might be thoughts that you've had or words someone has said to you. However, these beliefs came into your life, they run deep. They are walls getting in your way of the one thing you want most, to become a family.

Sometimes these walls feel impossible to climb, and that only deepens these beliefs. The thought spirals can be terrifying:

"If getting pregnant is the one thing you want most in the world, then how on earth can you not lose a bit of weight to achieve it? Losing weight is easy right?

Respecting your body

Just eating the right foods and exercising, so why can't you do something so simple? Obviously, you don't want to be a mother enough if you can't do this simple thing. Obviously, you are not worthy enough of being a mother if you can't even lose a bit of weight."

It's an endless spiral of hatred towards yourself and your body. So instead of going into this downward spiral, will you join me on an upward spiral instead? What if it was not only possible to get pregnant when you're fat, but it was easy? What if you were good enough to be a mother exactly how you are. Right this minute. What if you didn't have to change a thing to get pregnant?

How does that make you feel? It's freeing, right? The conditions that are stopping you from getting pregnant may be in your head. No, I don't mean you are going crazy, and I'm not belittling everything you are experiencing as trivial right now. This is a good thing. This is the **positive** part of the FAT+ve framework. Creating a positive set of beliefs and thoughts is a powerful way to impact your health in all aspects positively.

Every single thing that happens in your life, no matter how big or small, is just a thing. It isn't good or bad, it's an external circumstance. We, as human beings, give everything meaning based on our existing beliefs about the world.

So all those beliefs you have (whether you know you have them or not) are colouring the world in which you live. You are making decisions and taking action based on that data which is positively skewed to match your current belief system.

If you think you are a lucky person, you will naturally see the world through a filter where lucky things happen to you. You will take opportunities believing that a positive outcome will follow. Things happen, but the meaning we give them, that happens in our head. And from there, our body responds accordingly.

A meeting with your boss is just a thing. But when you put that meeting through your internal filters, you may think this is a bad thing, maybe you're worried about a mistake you made at work or that they're laying people off. You've applied that meaning to the thing based on your experiences and your beliefs. Your body will now respond. Your body will go into a stressed state. Your heart will beat faster, your blood will pump quicker around your body, and you will breathe more quickly. All because you assigned meaning to a situation.

Over time, being in a chronically stressed state may lead to IBS (Irritable Bowel Syndrome), migraines, insomnia and a whole host of other conditions that we live within this day and age. And all this stems from our head. It's all in our mind. Do you know what the great thing about this is? We have the power to change it. Your thoughts and beliefs are entirely changeable. You can choose them every second of every day. Mind-blowing, right?

You can choose to believe that you are good enough to be a mother right now. You can choose to believe that fat makes no difference to whether you get pregnant or now. You can choose to be completely confident in whatever you decide to wear. It can take a little time for these beliefs to become second nature (or maybe I could believe that new thoughts come to me easily!!!!) and you do need to be vigilant in your thoughts, but the benefits are endless.

You can create the life of your dreams from this simple method. So right now I want you to choose to be good enough right now, exactly as you are.

How to find self-compassion

So you've said to yourself a few times, I'm good enough, I believe in myself, I'm worthy enough to be a mother. Now what? How can you filter these sentiments into your everyday life so that they become a part of who you are?

Without weaving them into the fabric of you, they are just nice sentiments. Something nice to say to yourself, even if you don't really believe it. So let's get working these into the fabric of your very being.

Whenever we, as humans, create a belief around something, we look for evidence. Not in a very scientific way, more in an extremely biased "what can I use to back up what I already believe" kinda way.

Say, for example, your mum told you that whenever a black cat crossed your path, something terrible was about to happen to you. All of a sudden, a black cat has meaning. You notice when you see a black cat (much more than any other coloured cat), and if something terrible happened a few minutes/hours/days after you saw the cat, it would be "evidence" that your mother was right and black cats were evil. But what happens if a tabby cat crosses your path? And what about all the times a black cat crossed your path and nothing happened? You don't remember these things because they didn't back up your belief. It's a positive bias for what you already believe.

Your brain actively does this without you even realising. Confirming what it already knows. So how can we use this to our advantage?

Let's take the example "you are good enough right now exactly as you are". What evidence can you find to help you back up this statement? Let's start with the basics.

If you are reading this, I can pretty much guarantee you've kept yourself alive for this long. No matter what life has thrown at you, no matter what circumstances you've found yourself in, you've managed to pull yourself through to get to this moment in time. Think back to all the shit you've had to deal with, all the crap life has thrown at you and all the seemingly impossible situations you've come out of the other side of. You've done pretty bloody well to get here now.

The final biggie is getting pregnant. Sometimes it can feel like your body is public enemy number one. It goes out of its way to throw a spanner in the works, with its crazy cycles, irritating symptoms and basically doing everything it can to annoy you while stopping you from having the thing you want most in the world.

But that's not really what is happening. Your body is trying to talk to you. It started off as a whisper, but the longer it went without being heard, the louder it had to shout for us to take notice. In our society, we are used to taking a magic pill to fix things, but we don't really ever get to the root of what caused the problem in the first place. Got a headache? Take a pain killer, but what caused the headache?

Your body is actually looking out for you by not getting pregnant. Stay with me here. If you're going through some health stuff (whatever that stuff may be), then it may be really bloody hard on your body to get pregnant. If you are chronically stressed then your body thinks that you are in a life or death situation (it doesn't know the difference between a drought and a busy time at work) it's going to put off the whole bringing new life into the world.

The Guilt

The guilt of being fat is overwhelming in our society. In a culture where fat is blamed for every health issue, every symptom, every problem, it's easy to see why we all feel so guilty. After all, we are made to believe that being fat is our fault, a character flaw. We are greedy. We are lazy. There is something wrong with us because we cannot be or stay thin just like society wants.

That's when the guilt starts to kick in. Because it should be easy to lose weight. Everyone says how easy it is. Just stick to this simple plan. How hard can it be? And if it's so easy, then there is most definitely something wrong with you. And it's all your fault.

Except it's not. It's not your fault that the food industry values its sales more than your health. It's not your fault that an unhealthy body ideal is all we see in our constant stream of media everywhere we look. It's not your fault that the diet industry only works if it keeps us dieting, and that means losing then putting the weight back on.

I may sound cynical, but it's the truth. These things are working against you in more ways than you realise. Think about it in a different way - if you loved your body and accepted it exactly as it was. If everyone did this....

There would be no beauty industry, no fashion industry, no cosmetic surgery.
Every industry that bases its marketing on making us feel less than so that they can sell us products that make us feel better about ourselves would be out of business. But let's face it, we aren't going to change these industries overnight, so where do we start? How can we get comfortable with this guilt we feel about not being able to get pregnant? Not being able to eat the "right" foods, not being our healthiest self for our future baby?

The first thing we need to do is take the pressure off and take away all those shoulds. Anything you start with "I should do this........" has gotta go.

Exercise

This is a fun one! I want you to make a list of all the things you do in your life. I know, I know, sounds overwhelming already but just start and see what comes up. Set a timer for 15mins and just use whatever comes up in that time

Grab a pen and paper or download the "Fat and Fertile" accompanying PDF that contains all the exercises from the book that you can fill in straight on your computer or print off.

Access the PDF at nicolasalmon.co.uk/bookbonus

Be a general or a specific as you want.

Then I want you to grab some coloured pens.
Any activities that feel restful mark in one colour - this could be sleep (hopefully!) reading hobbies walking anything that feels rejuvenating

Any activities that feel playful mark in another colour

With the rest of the activities - really think about how important they are.

If they are essential - how can you bring more play or rest to them

If they are non-essential, can you get rid of them or get someone else to do them?

I'd love to know what you uncover in this exercise, share your ahas on Instagram hashtag #fatandfertile or email me nicola@nicolasalmon.co.uk.

So what exactly do you feel guilty about?

Being fat - what can you do about this right now? Check in with your body. How does being fat feel physically to you? Are you in any pain? The majority of the guilt comes from worrying about what other people are thinking about us. Worrying about other people's opinions used to make sense when we needed our tribe to protect us, but the world doesn't work that way anymore.

Eating food you've labelled as bad - you can choose to make healthier choices, but it's a choice. "Bad" food isn't bad. We are always hearing on the news about the latest food that scientists labelled bad but are now good?

It's time to take away the useless labels and look at the real reasons we are eating what we are eating. Is the chocolate going to help you feel better in your mental health? There is a reason for everything we do. Take a little time to figure out your reason.

Not being pregnant - this is the worst one. You can feel like you're letting down your family, letting down your partner and letting down yourself. The illusion is that it's all your fault that you aren't pregnant. That it's your body that isn't working as it should so it must be your fault. But once we strip away the illusion that a) being fat is unhealthy and b) being fat is your fault. We can see that the fat on your body has nothing to do with it.

Whatever decisions you made in the past, you did the best you could with what you knew. It's time to forgive your past self. She was trying her hardest to keep you going. To live in a world which is bloody difficult at times. She did the best she possibly could.

What can present you do? Thinking only about today, what ways can you feel good and really look after your body and your mind?

Leave the rest for your future self to worry about. All we have to focus on is today.

Exercise

It's time to forgive your body for not being pregnant and for every other mistake it's made.

Grab a pen and paper and write down every negative experience you've had with your body.

Some ideas:

Start from your head and work down each part of your body. If something comes up, write it down.
Think about any tests, operations or illnesses you've ever had
Think about any times people have made fun of you for what you look like

Once you've got the list. Go through each bullet point and repeat the following
Take a deep breath
Feel the emotion you felt at the time

> Say out loud or in your head "I forgive you. I'm sorry. Thank you. I love you."
>
> Repeat for every point.

How to treat your body with respect

When you've decided that weight loss isn't the way to go, it can feel alien. It's a free and scary place all at once. The unknown territory can feel lonely, and it can be tempting to run straight back to what feels comfortable and safe.

We are so used to blaming our body for everything that is going wrong, that we have no clue how to treat it when we aren't at war with it. We're being told over and over that it is our bodies fault. After all, your body isn't playing ball. It's not regulating your hormones in the way it should, maybe you've been diagnosed with Endometriosis, PCOS, a blocked tube, premature ovarian failure, even if the doctors have found no cause, it must be your bodies fault right? If everything was working in your body, you'd be able to get pregnant with ease.

But that's not the whole story. As a fat woman, I've spent my life believing my body wasn't good enough. That I was less than because my body didn't look like the pictures in the magazines. I didn't believe that I was worthy of love, worthy of becoming a wife or a mother.

But I am. I was born worthy, and so were you. You do not have to achieve any goal, be a particular body type or change anything about you to be worthy of being a mother.

Your body is sacred. Your body is going to create life and carry that life for nine months until your baby is ready to enter the world. No matter what you believe, that truly is a miracle, and your body deserves to be treated with respect and nourished to be ready for that miracle. It's time! It's time to step up and treat your body with the respect that it deserves. Not when you're pregnant. Not when you're skinnier. NOW.

I know that after reading this chapter, you are going to be fired up. You are going to want to take some action and take it now! You've wasted too much time already listening to others over you. You've been lied to for too long about what your body needs and what you need. So what can you do right now to start treating your body with respect?

I've got seven things you can start to do today. Right now. Pick one, the one that hits you square in the face when you read it. That's the one.

There is one important point before you get started, though. I don't want you to do it perfectly. I don't want you to make this into another stick to beat yourself up with. Each of these things can be done slowly, imperfectly and with kindness.

This is the start of the process. It's not about getting to the end as quickly as possible. There is no end. It's about being curious, making mistakes and finding what feels good for you. Tag me on Instagram @fatpositivefertility with your favourite step and show me how you are finding ways to make you feel good.

Buy clothes that fit your body
Don't buy clothes to aspire to, ones that you hope to fit in when you've lost weight. Don't buy the first thing that fits, just because you can no longer bear the pain of clothes shopping. Buy clothes that make you feel amazing. Buy underwear that looks great (goodbye 10-year-old granny pants!). Buy clothes

that fit your body perfectly. You deserve to feel comfortable in your clothes each and every day.

Nourish your body with food that makes it feel good.

Choose food that gives you energy (the good kind, not the rollercoaster kind), that makes you feel good. Eat mindfully, notice how the food tastes, how hungry or full you feel, how you feel when you eat it. Infuse your food with love and the intention that this food is going to make your body strong and healthy.

Move your body in a way that feels good

Your body is designed to move every day. Find movement that brings you joy. Find ways to fit it easily into your life.

Prioritise your self-care

Self-care is not just bubble baths and spa days. It's the act of choosing yourself each and every day, above everyone else. Choosing to put your needs first. It isn't selfish. You can only help others when you are replenished. Think about what your needs are and ensure that you find a way to meet them every day.

Pay attention to your thoughts

You have been bullying your body for a long time. Telling it that it's useless, that it's ugly, that it's unworthy of anything. It's time for that to stop. Pay attention to the thoughts you are thinking and the language you are using every day about your body. First, spend some time noticing it. Then every time you notice that you are using negative language, say in your head, "STOP, this is not useful" and flip it. If you were thinking "my tummy is so fat and ugly" say instead "my tummy is beautiful and soft" even if you don't believe it. This is a practice so keep practising.

Give your body enough sleep

Sleep is vital for every aspect of our health. Sleep is for the strong, not the weak. You need to prioritise it. Ensure that you are getting at least 8 hours each night. Keep all electronics out of the bedroom. Avoid blue light (phones, tv, laptops) at least 30min before bed. Keep an eye on what caffeine and alcohol are doing to your body. If you struggle with sleep, get some help.

Check out of the diet culture talk

Talk about weight loss, bikini bodies and unrealistic beauty standards is everywhere. It's difficult to escape it, but if you want to create a loving relationship with your body, there is no room for that negativity in your life. Do not be available for that kind of crap from anyone. Unfollow anyone on social media who promotes that. Avoid newspapers, magazines and websites that promise you can lose 2 stone in 2 weeks. Change the subject with friends, family and work colleagues when these topics come up or if you feel brave enough, tell them that you are no longer interested in talking about these things anymore.

Can you respect your fat body?

When you have been trying to lose weight your whole adult life, and you've been told that you have to lose weight to get pregnant, it can feel impossible to go against that.

The simple facts are these: Diets don't work. The research that shows that a higher BMI equates with higher infertility, higher risks in pregnancy and higher risks for baby are hugely flawed. You are capable of having a healthy pregnancy and a healthy baby in your fat body.

Respecting your body

I want you to choose you. Every day when you wake up, I want you to make a decision to live your life in the best way you can right now. Being fertile isn't some uber health goal we need to "level-up" to. Your fertility is a reflection of your health, so working on what is going to make you feel healthier and happier is the best way to improve your ability to get pregnant.

So what do you think? Can you really learn to respect a fat body?

Exercise

Grab a pen and paper. One one side I want you to write down the names of your 5 favourite people.

Got it? And beside each person I want you to write down the 3 things you love about them. So 15 things in total.

On the other side, I want you to draw a picture of you. Don't worry if you aren't an artist, a stick person is great. You can spend as little or as much time as you want on this, draw the you that you see in the mirror.
Beside your picture I want you to write 15 things that you love about yourself.

Now compare the lists.

On each list, you have 15 things. The first list describes all the things you love about your favourite people. These are characteristics and traits that you love in the people you choose to have in your life.

The second list details all the things you love about you.

What do you notice between the two lists? Are they similar at all? How do they differ?

I'm going to bet that the things you love about your favourite people are more about how they treat you and how they make you feel rather than what they look like.

What's on the list of things you love about you? Are they nice sentiments? Things that it's ok to like about yourself - you're generous, caring of others, nice, kind….. blah blah blah they are all well and good, but they say nothing about the real you.

How many physical attributes did you list? Did you only pick the "socially acceptable" things you are allowed to like about your fat body? Your eyes, your hair, your lips - all things that aren't affected by your fat.

But what about your gorgeous breasts? Your incredible strong legs? Your beautiful, soft and squishy tummy? We have been told we are not allowed to enjoy these things about our body, that they are bad and unworthy of our love for them.

So back to those lists. What things do you love about yourself and your body that really make you who you are? Forget which parts please others. Maybe you love your cutting sense of humour, your eclectic sense of style, your photographic memory?

Let's embrace the things about us that are unapologetically us! Not the niceties that please everyone, the difficult, brilliant, the uncomfortable and the different.

Respecting your body

Here are some things that I really love about me:

- My willingness to cancel things at the last minute if I need to look after myself more
- When I let my armpit hair grow - it feels so soft and fluffy
- My confidence when I'm naked and feel great in my own skin
- My unwillingness to compromise on things I'm really passionate about
- My bloody-minded stubbornness not to give up on the really important things
- My Mary Poppins like abilities with small children (except my own)
- My capacity to give love to anyone who needs it.

You don't have to do this all in one go. Right now, it feels safe to stay within the social norms, to follow the crowd and to do what everyone else is doing. There is a reason for that. In ye olde times, if you were different or weird, the risks were much higher. You could be shunned and cast out from your tribe, and without that protection, you'd probably die alone. There are evolutionary reasons why we try to fit in and want to be liked so much.

But that isn't a big enough reason to spend your whole time hating your body. Trust me, there are far better things you can be doing with your time.

And as for a fat body that can't get pregnant? Your body is doing it's absolute best to protect you. Your body is here for you. If you are hating on it and punishing it and feeling disgusted about it, it doesn't think its the right time for baby making. So the best thing you can do is to start to be kind to it in every way you know how. Whisper it loving words, feed it nourishing foods, move it with passion and above all treat it like you would your best friend.

I saw a great video the other day about an experiment that some kids did in their school. They got two identical plants and put them in identical conditions.

They put a sign above each one. The first instructed the students to treat this plant with love, send it loving thoughts, give it compliments and treat it nicely. The second sign told the students to bully the plant. Send it cruel thoughts and tell the plant how rubbish it was. Remarkably there was a huge difference between how the plants grew. Kindness really did help the plant to grow.

Obviously, this is not a scientific experiment, and I'm sure there are plenty of other "normal" explanations for why this happened. But it makes you think, right? If you are bombarding your body each and every day with negative thoughts, what is that doing to your cells, your organs, your brain? How is it impacting on your mood and your happiness?

So today I want you to take one step to find a way to love your body, like your body or even just accepting that you want to learn to love your body. Maybe it's throwing away all the baggy, hole-ridden misshapen clothes in your wardrobe and wearing clothes that fit and make you look great. While you're at it, you can get rid of (or at least pack away) all the clothes that are 2 sizes too small or 2 sizes too big. Maybe you are going to cancel your gym membership and find a form of exercise that makes you feel amazing and that lights you up every time you do it. Maybe you want to begin to explore what foods really nourish your body, regardless of how many calories or grams of fat they have in them.

Every step you take towards loving your body more will take you one step closer to creating the perfect environment for your baby.

Chapter 9 - What happens when I get pregnant?

I've been a fat mama for five years now. What they say is true - the days are long but the years are short. I still can't believe my eldest is at school. I was worried about being a fat mother, but yet again, most of these fears come from worrying about what other people would think of me.

- Will they think I'm a bad mum that feeds her kids junk food?
- Will they think my children are going to be unhealthy?
- Will they think I'm irresponsible for having kids when I'm fat?
- Will I make no mum friends and my child never been invited to play dates and parties?

Some of these sound silly, but for me, they felt (and still sometimes do) feel very real. I actually got trolled a little while ago on Instagram.

"If you want to be fat, fine. But don't subject your kids to the same fate" was what someone wrote on one of my posts.

Jaw drop!!!! This was another mother - who I have never met or had any contact with. This was a big learning moment. My first thought was "has she seen my kids?" Erm, definitely both very healthy and happy weights.

Second thought - WTF? Why am I even thinking that? What if they were fat? It's not of her fucking business!

Third thought - My work is actually around helping women heal their relationship with food and their bodies. There is no room in my universe for judging or shaming humans. PERIOD!

Final thought (for now!) Deep breath - No room for judgement includes this woman - forgive and let it go. This stuff sometimes tangles me in knots and that's ok. We are all unlearning years of this stuff.

A huge worry I had was about passing on my negative self-confidence and issues around food to my kids.

This was one of the reasons I stopped dieting and weighing myself. I realised that kids just copy what you do. No amount of talking to them about food and their bodies in a healthy way would do any good if I wasn't showing them with my actions.

It's also a huge reason why I do this work. Imagine if every fat woman loved her body and had a really healthy relationship with food. These incredible women would model this to their children (who now come easily because they no longer believe that their weight is a barrier to pregnancy) who grow up loving their bodies, filled with self-acceptance and an understanding that the food they eat does not reflect their self-worth. A generation of change makers, can you imagine it?

Now that my boys are past the baby stage, I've been contemplating what kind of mama I want to be. Not what shape I wanted my body to be, but how I want to show up in their lives, how I want us to spend time together as a family. I knew instantly that I wanted to be an active mama. For so long "active = skinny" in my head, so it took a big leap in my mindset to start to believe that I was going to move my body for the reason of making me feel good.

What happens when I get pregnant?

Every single time I leave the house to exercise, I make the decision to choose to move my body because it makes me feel good. And it does! The most profound result of regular exercise for me has been regular periods. My periods went from 100+ days to between 30-40. Still not super consistent but way better than before. This change did not coincide with weight loss. My body is still the same size, but the decision I took for my health was real.

Researchers have known since the 1970s that diets do not work long term and cause weight to regain. The diet industry does not want you to know that so guess what? They sponsor research in the field and "support" governments to battle the "obesity epidemic".

Your body does not need an external voice telling it what it needs to eat. Your body is perfectly capable of giving you that information. You can trust your body to support your health and fertility. We just have to learn to listen again.

We've explored the real reasons why the risks increase for women in bigger bodies exists when you want to get pregnant. But when you do get pregnant, these reasons don't go away.

Looking at the big picture, it's easy to see why the risks increase with the size of the patient's body. It is nothing to do with the amount of fat that they have around their middle and everything to do with the bias they face every day and the extreme dieting and exercise we are coerced into doing to live in our society.

But these risks are avoidable. And not by artificially controlling your weight for a period of time. We can choose to support and nourish our bodies with food in the way that they need. We can choose foods that make our bodies feel good, and that gives us energy and help us sleep.

We can listen to our bodies cues and eat foods that we crave. We can honour our bodies choices. You can learn more about this by reading "Intuitive Eating" by Elyse Resch and Evelyn Tribole or by enrolling on The Fertility UnDiet course, an 8-week course to support you in learning how to listen to your body again around food.

We can also choose our healthcare team with intention. If we are in a position to, we can choose doctors who won't shame us and tell us to "just lose some weight", we can educate our healthcare team in our boundaries and our needs.

Slowly but surely we can erode away the old system where the doctor would tell the patient what to do, and the patient would follow blindly. Instead, we can be part of a team where we are encouraged to make our own choices for our bodies and the doctors provide their recommendations based on science and their own experience, through a lens of respect for every individual.

Fat pregnancy

But the conversation doesn't end once you are pregnant. When I got pregnant with both my boys, I was lumped into a category of "high risk" based purely on the weighing scales. All my other health indicators were normal.

This had an impact on how I was monitored throughout my pregnancy and the birth choices I was given. Thankfully this was also the cue for me to begin to research around my own healthcare rights. I knew that I wanted a water birth at home, but I was informed that this wasn't an option as I was high risk. I did a lot of research into this area, and it was the first time I ever stood up against healthcare professionals advice and asked for what I wanted. It was the first time that I realised that maybe my doctor didn't have all the information. That the decisions they were making on behalf of my health weren't based on all the facts.

What happens when I get pregnant?

It was such an empowering moment for me to "make a fuss" and use the evidence I had found to insist that this was what I wanted. And they weren't able to say no because it was my choice. And this information just blew my mind. I was so used to doing what I was told. I was a good girl through and through. I went out of my way to make sure that others were happy, anticipating their needs, not making a fuss, afraid to take up space.

A typical (yet completely ridiculous) example of this was when I went to my boyfriends (now husbands) parents house for the first time. Of course, as a guest, they asked me what I wanted to drink, and I said "nothing, I'm fine thanks" My boyfriend looked at me questioningly, like "really?" Such a simple act opened my eyes. I had no idea if I wanted a drink. "No thanks, I'm fine" automatically came out of my mouth before I even had time to decide if I wanted a drink. Because I didn't want to put them out. Because I didn't want to make a fuss. In my head, the simple act of getting me a drink was too much to ask.

Then I started to see this pattern everywhere. I moved out of everyone's way as I walked down the street. I worried about my bag on the seat of the bus as soon as other people got on. Whenever anyone asked me what I wanted to do or which restaurant I wanted to eat at, my answer was always "I don't mind".

I used to think it's because I was easy going, but I realise now it's because I didn't value myself. I didn't think I was worthy enough of having my needs met, of making my opinion known. I don't think I'm alone in this. I see it in my sister every time I ask her what she wants for lunch.

I recently read an article my friend Charlotte wrote about a game she likes to call Patriarchy Chicken. It basically involves her walking around busy London and not moving aside when men are walking towards her. She has been bumped into a lot!

As women, we have been taught to be the good girl. We have been taught to put others above ourselves, and even in this day and age, we have been led to believe that others have rights to make decisions over our bodies which they definitely do not!

If you are able to, when you get pregnant (and my love, that is totally possible for you in your current body, and you are worthy of that right now) find a doctor who will not shame you during your pregnancy.

Here are some great women who are creating resources for pregnant women in larger bodies:

Jen McLellan at Plus Mommy[14]
Amber Marshall at Big Birthas[15]
Pamela Vireday at Well Rounded Mama[16]

If you aren't able to get a doctor who supports you fully, create clear boundaries in your relationship. What is ok for you? What isn't ok for you? You are well within your rights to ask not to be weighed at every appointment and if weighing is essential for you not to see that number if it is triggering for you. You are allowed to tell your doctor that you are not willing to discuss diets and other "lifestyle" factors. You are allowed to be difficult and demanding and stubborn, and all the other things that "good girls" aren't allowed to be.

You are allowed to accept nothing less than unbiased, patient-centred, respectful healthcare. And the more people that demand this level of care, the more that it will be given.

---

[14] https://plusmommy.com

[15] http://bigbirthas.co.uk

[16] https://wellroundedmama.blogspot.com

What happens when I get pregnant?

Our children (yes, yours too) will never have to feel that shame of being made to feel that their body wasn't good enough. They will grow up with confidence in their bodies and a healthy relationship with food. Our daughters will be respected for their gifts and not just seen as their bodies. Our sons will stand up for those marginalised around them. The next generation will stand for better treatment of all.

It starts with us, here, now, with as much emotional energy as we are able to give, asking for what is rightfully ours. Equal healthcare.

No matter what happens during your future pregnancy, it is not your fault. Whether you have a healthy pregnancy or experience some common pregnancy issues, your body is not to blame. As much as we'd like to believe that making healthy choices all the time means that we are going to stay healthy, that's not how health works.

Illness does not limit itself to the unhealthy. There are so many factors about our health that are out of our control, and as soon as we realise that these things can and do happen at random, we can stop blaming ourselves for everything.

Every bad thing that has happened to you is not because you are fat. You didn't deserve those things because you don't look the way our society has dictated to us. This is evidence that the risks of particular conditions during pregnancy are elevated, but that does not mean that they happen to every pregnant fat person. These risks should be discuss in an non-bias, and non-shaming way and you should be allowed to decide what is acceptable risk for you.

In the book "Politics of Size" edited by Ragen Chastain, Pamela Vireday writes in her essay "New Frontiers in Weight Bias: The Womb as Ground Zero in the War on Obesity", that news articles rarely place the risks associated with their sensationalist headlines in any context. She goes on to say that "if they did, readers would see that, although at increased risk for some things, *most* fat women do not experience the given particular complication."

Vireday explains further in her blog post "Exaggerating the Risks Again"[17] that the 2-4 x risk for birth defects in women with bigger bodies is still a very small risk. The risk for Neural Tube Defects is still less than 1%, meaning that 99% of women in bigger bodies with not have a baby with a Neural Tube Defect.

The risks are also distorted for diabetes and high blood pressure complications. Vireday states that:

"Weiss (AJOG, 2004), a large study of more than 16,000 women in multiple hospital centers, found that 9.5% of "morbidly obese" women (BMI more than 35) experienced Gestational Diabetes during their study. The number certainly is higher than the 2.3% with a BMI less than 30, so it is definitely a risk (*4x the risk---gasp!*) that should be communicated to women of size.

However, it also means that 90% of "morbidly obese" women did *not* develop Gestational Diabetes. So while the risk increased, it should be remembered that the vast majority of morbidly obese women will *not* get GD.

Pre-eclampsia is another risk that is substantially increased in "obese" women, and this one can be life-threatening to both mother and baby. It is definitely a risk that must be discussed as a possibility and taken very seriously. But in the Weiss study, only 6.3% of "morbidly obese" women developed Pre-eclampsia....higher than the 2.1% of non-obese women (*3.3x the risk---gasp!*) who developed PE, but hardly universal. Remember, 93% of "morbidly obese" women did *not* develop Pre-eclampsia in that study.

---

[17]wellroundedmama.blogspot.com

Again, the majority of these women did *not* get GD or PE, the two most common risks for women of size.

So while these risks *are* real and it's only sensible that the possibility be discussed with women of size (and that women of size be proactive about lessening their risk for them), it's important that the magnitude of the risks not be exaggerated or to imply that such a complication is virtually inevitable."

The risks are present, but it does not mean that being fat is causing these conditions. If this were true, all women in bigger bodies would get diabetes and pre-eclampsia. Vireday suggests that "Another possible theory is that underlying metabolic differences is really behind these complications, and the fatness is merely a byproduct of these metabolic differences, a *symptom* if you will.

Making the women diet will likely not help much unless the underlying metabolic differences are also addressed. Trying to fix things by losing large amounts of weight is too simplistic an approach."

And what about being a fat mother?

I think this was the very last idea that I had to let go of. I thought getting pregnant would be the ultimate motivator for losing weight. I tried (and failed) for my wedding. But kids are different, right? I want to be the best mother I could be and in my head that involved being active, which of course equalled thin.

This thought led me down all sorts of merry paths. If I can't lose weight, then obviously I don't want to be a mum enough? If I don't lose weight, then I won't be a very good mother? What if my kids get teased because of me?

Nicola Salmon

I've got good news from the other side.

I am a fantastic mother, and I have a fat body. My mothering is not affected by my size. My boys love me absolutely unconditionally. They love my big tummy and blow raspberries on it regularly which they find absolutely hilarious!

They don't even give my body a second thought because I'm their mama and that's all that matters. They won't love me any more or less if my weight changes. The incredible thing about being a mama in a fat body is being able to learn with them how we respect our bodies and all other bodies. About how bodies come in all shapes and sizes and that it's completely normal. We talk about periods, about gender fluidity, about consent.

This incredible journey back to my own body has allowed me to model that new found respect for them. Very early on, I told them that they didn't have to kiss/hug anyone that they didn't want to. I wanted to show them what consent looked like from the beginning and that they had full control over their bodies. I used the phrase "your body, your choice" often.

It's come back to bite me in the bum now, as anytime I ask them to do anything it's "my body, my choice" but I hope that it is going to stand them in good stead for the future.

Conclusion

I hope reading this book has given you a new found respect for your body and opened the door to see what your body is capable of. You are capable of creating miracles right now and you are so worthy of those miracles. No matter what has happened in the past, you deserve to become a parent and be supported in that desire.

The road ahead may appear long and difficult but I promise that by using the tools in this book, putting one foot in front of the other and prioritising you every day, you will reach your goal and somehow you will become the epic parent you know that you were born to be. The route may not always look how you pictured but I promise you that by trusting your gut and following the breadcrumbs on your path, you will get (and already are) exactly where you need to be.

If you need some more support or want to find out more about my work, you can follow me on Instagram or Facebook @fatpositivefertility or join my weekly-ish newsletter via my website www.nicolasalmon.co.uk

A great way to support my work and get even more tools to make this experience easier is to join my Fat Positive Fertility Hub. The resources and tools are organised into the four key areas of the Fat Positive Fertility Framework. Simply chose the area you want to focus on first and use the resources to build your toolkit. Each month a new resource will be added to the hub. There is a small monthly investment because I believe that investing in your health is an act of love. It sets the intention that you are willing to commit to working on this process. I want to model how important it is to honour yourself. So often we, as women, are expected to be selfless and give ourselves unconditionally to others without asking for anything in return. It is so important that together we start asking for a return on the physical and emotional labour we undertake for the people around us. And by investing a small amount each month, you are supporting my work so that I can continue to fight for our right to fertility support in the healthcare system.

If you want to go deeper, I take on a small number of 1-1 clients from all over the world to support them with their goal of getting pregnant in a fat body. Email me nicola@nicolasalmon.co.uk for more details.

But the one thing that I want you to take away from this book my love, is that it's OK for you to want to become a parent. You are not alone. You are not selfish or irresponsible. You should not be made to feel ashamed or guilty. You should not be judged for your body.

You are just a parent waiting for their child.

Further Reading

• Adams, Louise, and Willer, Fiona, *Everything You've Been Told About Weight Loss is Bullshit* (e-book accessed at https://dietingisbs.carrd.co/, 2017)

• Bacon, Linda, *Health At Every Size: The Surprising Truth About Your Weight* (BenBella Books 2010)

• Bacon, Linda, and Aphramor, Lucy, *Body Respect: What Conventional Health Books Get Wrong, Leave Out, and Just Plain Fail to Understand about Weight* (BenBella Books, 2014)

• Baker, Jess, *Landwhale: on Turning Insults Into Nicknames, Why Body Image is Hard, and How Diets Can Kiss My Ass* (Seal Press, 2018)

• Baker, Jess, *Things No One Will Tell Fat Girls* (Seal Press, 2015)

• Chastain, Ragen, *The Politics of Size: Perspectives from the Fat Acceptance Movement* (Praeger, 2015)

• Crabbe, Megan Jayne, *Body Positive Power: How to stop dieting, make peace with your body and live* (Vermilion, 2017)

• Dooner, Caroline, *The F*ck It Diet: Eating Should be Easy* (Harper Collins UK, 2019)

• Elman, Michelle, *Am I Ugly?* (Anima, 2018)

• Hagen, Sofie, *Happy Fat: Taking Up Space in a World That Wants to Shrink You* (Harper Collins UK, 2019)

- Harrison, Christy, *Anti-Diet: Reclaim Your Time, Money, Well-Being, and Happiness Through Intuitive Eating* (Hachette UK, 2020)[18]

- Sole-Smith, Virginia, *The Eating Instinct: Food Culture, Body Image and Guilt in America* (Henry Holt and Company, 2018)

- Taylor, Sonya Renee, *The Body is Not an Apology: The Power of Radical Self-Love* (Berrett-Koehler, 2018)

- Thomas, Laura, *Just Eat It: How intuitive eating can help you get your shit together around food* (Bluebird, 2019)

- Tovar, Virgie, *You Have the Right to Remain Fat* (Melvin House UK, 2018)

- Tribal, Evelyn, and Resch, Elyse, *Intuitive Eating: A Revolutionary Program that Works* (Revised ed. Edition: Griffin, 2012)

---

[18] Anti-Diet isn't out yet when this book is published but I'm including it because I know it's going to be amazing!

Made in the USA
Coppell, TX
05 June 2020